Learning About AIDS

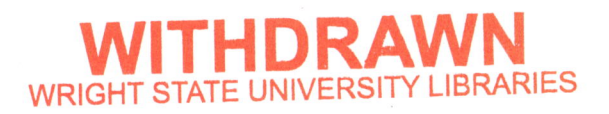

*This book is dedicated to the memory
of
Simon Mansfield*

*who pioneered the development
of high quality treatment
and care services in the community
for people with HIV*

For Churchill Livingstone

Commissioning Editor: Mary Law
Project Editor: Valerie Bain
Senior Project Controller: Neil A. Dickson
Project Controller: Nicola S. Haig
Copy Editor: Jennifer Bew
Design: Judith Wright
Sales Promotion Executive: Hilary Brown

Learning About AIDS
Scientific and Social Issues

Edited by

Peter Aggleton
Kim Rivers
Ian Warwick
Geoff Whitty

Health and Education Research Unit
Institute of Education
University of London

SECOND EDITION

Published in association with the Health Education Authority

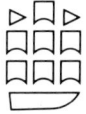

CHURCHILL LIVINGSTONE
EDINBURGH LONDON MADRID MELBOURNE NEW YORK AND TOKYO 1994

CHURCHILL LIVINGSTONE
Medical Division of Longman Group Limited

Distributed in the United States of America by Churchill Livingstone Inc.,
650 Avenue of the Americas, New York, N.Y. 10011, and by associated companies, branches and representatives throughout the world.

© Peter Aggleton, Hilary Homans, Jan Mojsa, Stuart Watson, Simon Watney 1989
© Longman Group Limited 1994

All rights reserved. No part of this publication may be reproduced, stored in a retrieval system, or transmitted in any form or by any means, electronic, mechanical, photocopying, recording or otherwise, without either the prior permission of the publishers (Churchill Livingstone, Robert Stevenson House, 1–3 Baxter's Place, Leith Walk, Edinburgh EH1 3AF), or a licence permitting restricted copying in the United Kingdom issued by the Copyright Licensing Agency Ltd, 90 Tottenham Court Road, London, W1P 9HE.

First edition 1989 (Peter Aggleton, Hilary Homans, Jan Mojsa, Stuart Watson, Simon Watney)
Second edition 1994 (Longman Group Limited)

ISBN 0 443 05178 X

British Library Cataloguing in Publication Data
A catalogue record for this book is available from the British Library.

Library of Congress Cataloging in Publication Data
Learning about AIDS : scientific and social issues / edited by Peter
    Aggleton... [et al.]. — 2nd ed.
        p.   cm.
    Rev. ed. of: AIDS, scientific and social issues. 1989.
    Includes bibliographical references and index.
    ISBN 0-443-05178-X
    1. AIDS (Disease)   2. AIDS (Disease)—Social aspects.
  I. Aggleton, Peter.   II. AIDS, scientific and social issues.
    [DNLM: 1. Acquired Immunodeficiency Syndrome.   2. HIV Infections.
  3. Health Education.   WD 308 L4375 1994]
  RC607.A26L423   1994
  362.1'969792—dc20
  DNLM/DLC
  for Library of Congress   94-16625

The publisher's policy is to use paper manufactured from sustainable forests

Printed in Great Britain by George Over Limited, Rugby and London

Contents

Contributors   vii

Preface   xi

1. Introduction   1
   Elaine Chase, Peter Aggleton

2. HIV and AIDS   13
   Edward King, Peter Scott, Peter Aggleton

3. Treatment and therapy   33
   Edward King, Peter Scott

4. Epidemiology, transmission and testing   53
   Simon Watney, Peter Aggleton

5. Sexual health   71
   Peter Aggleton, Paul Tyrer

6. HIV, AIDS and drug use   87
   Brian Pearson

7. Living with HIV and AIDS   97
   Peter Scott, Peter Aggleton, Paul Tyrer

References   115

Index   119

Contributors

Peter Aggleton is Co-Director of the Health and Education Research Unit, Institute of Education, University of London, and Reader in Education at Goldsmiths' College, University of London. He is currently on secondment to WHO, Geneva. He has worked extensively in HIV/AIDS health promotion. His publications include *Deviance* (Tavistock, 1987), *Social Aspects of AIDS* (Ed. with Hilary Homans, Falmer, 1988), *Health*, (Routledge, 1990), *AIDS: Responses, Interventions and Care* (Ed. with Graham Hart and Peter Davies, Falmer 1991), *AIDS: Rights, Risk and Reason* (Ed. with Peter Davies and Graham Hart, Falmer 1992) and *AIDS: Facing the Second Decade* (Ed. with Peter Davies and Graham Hart, Falmer, 1993).

Elaine Chase currently works and researches in southern Africa. Her interests are in the use of participatory research methods in the planning and management of health promotion with young women. She previously worked as a lecturer in health education at the Institute of Education, University of London.

Edward King is the Treatments Editor with the NAM Charitable Trust. From 1990 to 1992 he was Gay Men's Health Education Officer at the Terrence Higgins Trust in London. He is AIDS Editor of *The Pink Paper* and co-author (with Michael Rooney and Peter Scott) of *HIV Prevention with Gay and Bisexual Men: A survey of local initiatives* (North West Thames Regional Health Authority, 1992). He has written *Safety in Numbers* (Cassell, 1993), a study of gay men, safer sex and the 'de-gaying' of AIDS.

Brian Pearson is a freelance trainer and consultant specialising in drug and HIV issues. In the past he has worked for the Education Research Unit of Turning Point and the Standing Conference on Drug Abuse (SCODA). He was formerly HIV and Drugs Training Officer at the North West Regional Drug Training Unit. He is the author (with R. Griffiths) of *Working with Drug Users* (Wildwood, 1988), and of *Breaking the Connection*, a training and information book on drug use and HIV (Lifeline, 1991).

Kim Rivers was a research officer in the Health and Education Research Unit, Institute of Education, University of London. She is now a health education consultant at the College of Community Medicine, Lahore, Pakistan. She has co-authored a number of articles and training resources, including *AIDS: Working with Young People* (AVERT, 1993). She has taught health education in both the United States and the UK.

Peter Scott was editor of the *National AIDS Manual* until 1993. He is the founder of Gay Men Fighting AIDS. He is co-author (with Edward King and Michael Rooney) of *HIV Prevention with Gay and Bisexual Men: A survey of local initiatives* (North West Thames Regional Health Authority, 1992), and (with Michael Rooney) of *Developing Services for Gay Men and Bisexual Men* (Local Authority Associations' Officers Working Group on AIDS, 1993).

Paul Tyrer has been involved in HIV prevention work since 1987, including a spell as training and development officer on the HEA-funded Learning About AIDS project. He has also worked as an HIV/AIDS training officer both in the health service and the voluntary sector. He was joint coordinator of the Sheffield HIV Arts Festival 1992. He is currently carrying out research into the impact of HIV on gay men's writing at the University of Sheffield.

Simon Watney is Director of the Red Hot AIDS Charitable Trust, and has worked extensively in HIV/AIDS work in the UK and overseas since the early 1980s. He is the author of *Policing*

Desire: Pornography, AIDS and the Media (Minnesota, 1987), and co-editor with Erica Carter of *Taking Liberties: AIDS and Cultural Politics* (Serpent's Tail, 1989). His most recent book is *Practices of Freedom: Selected Writings on HIV/AIDS* (Rivers Oram, 1994). He has also been actively involved in sexual politics since Gay Liberation in 1971, and is a founder member of OutRage.

Ian Warwick is Assistant Director of the Health and Education Research Unit, Institute of Education, University of London. His publications include *AIDS: Working with Young People* (with Kim Rivers and Peter Aggleton, AVERT, 1993) and *Young People, Homelessness and HIV/AIDS Education* (Ed. with Peter Aggleton, Health Education Authority, 1992). His research interests are in professionals' perceptions of young people and informal sector care.

Geoff Whitty is Co-Director of the Health and Education Research Unit, Institute of Education, University of London, and Director of the Learning About AIDS project. He is also the Karl Mannheim Professor of Sociology of Education and Chair of the Department of Policy Studies at the Institute of Education.

Preface

The advent of HIV disease has created new priorities for those working in health education and health promotion. These include the need to clarify misunderstandings and allay fears and anxieties. The foundations for much of this have been laid through information campaigns, training and other educational activities in schools, at the workplace and in the community. Health educators in the health service, in local authorities and in voluntary organisations have a key role to play in such work, but need to be well prepared for the kinds of issues which can arise when helping others learn about HIV and AIDS. These include questions relating to scientific and medical matters, as well as individual and social responses to the epidemic.

Learning About AIDS: Scientific and Social Issues has been specially written with health educators in mind, regardless of whether they work in the health service, in local authorities or in voluntary organisations. It contains useful information on educational strategies, on the scientific and medical aspects of HIV and AIDS, on sexual behaviour and sexual health, on drug use, and on what it is like to live with HIV disease. Designed for use either on its own or as a preparation for health educators using the *Learning About AIDS** basic awareness training resource published by Churchill Livingstone, this book contains all the information needed to answer many of the questions likely to arise when educating people about HIV and AIDS.

The editors would like to thank Lyn Gorman and Helen Thomas for their assistance in producing this book. They would also like to acknowledge the support of Goldsmiths' College and the Institute of Education, University of London, which housed the Learning About AIDS project.

1994

P.A.
K.R.
I.W.
G.W.

Learning About AIDS: Training Guidance and Exercises (1994) by Peter Aggleton, Elaine Chase, Kim Rivers, Marilyn Toft, Paul Tyrer, Ian Warwick and Geoff Whitty is published by Churchill Livingstone in association with the Health Education Authority.

ical aspects of AIDS (acquired immune deficiency syn-
Introduction

Elaine Chase   Peter Aggleton

The physical aspects of AIDS (acquired immune deficiency syndrome) and HIV (human immunodeficiency virus) are now part of many people's lives and the broader social dimensions affect us all, even if this is not acknowledged by many. The World Health Organization's official figures state that at a conservative estimate 14 million infections had occurred worldwide by 1992 (WHO, 1993). Many of the people affected already have some of the symptoms and infections characteristic of HIV disease; some may have received a clinical diagnosis of AIDS. Yet others enjoy good health and have every chance of continuing to do so for some time, provided they have access to care and support services. In the UK, as elsewhere in the world, a large number of people are probably HIV antibody-positive and unaware of the fact. They may not consider themselves to have been at risk of exposure to the virus, or they may have decided not to determine their HIV status for a number of reasons. Fear of prejudice, stigma and discrimination all influence such decisions. Most strikingly, despite efforts to prevent further infection, there is every likelihood that many more people will become HIV antibody-positive in future.

The history of HIV now spans a complete decade, HIV having been identified as the virus responsible for AIDS in 1983. This period has witnessed a range of responses which have, at best, sought to empower and liberate, and at worst to control and oppress. Active and empowering movements which seek to provide appropriate information, advice and support for those with, or at risk from, HIV and AIDS are still largely the province of the voluntary sector and non-governmental organisations (NGOs). These are characteristic of the first responses to AIDS by gay men's organisations in the United States and Europe in the early 1980s. Besides their role in providing practical and psychological support for those already living with HIV and AIDS, such groups devised the notion of safer sex, thus developing a form of health education to which gay men and others affected in the epidemic could relate to minimise the risk of infection. Ten years on, the situation is very different. Most people now know something about AIDS and HIV and have some idea of how the virus is and is not transmitted. Yet, while statistics indicate a dramatic fall in the rate of new infections among gay men in the UK and elsewhere, since they have taken measures to minimise the risks, a progressive rise in the number of people with HIV who define themselves as heterosexual has simultaneously taken place and, worldwide, 90% of new HIV-positive test results are among heterosexuals (WHO, 1992a).

AIDS education is now the domain of many people, and recent years have seen a rapid increase in the number of new posts for HIV and AIDS specialists in statutory organisations, as well as in AIDS-specific voluntary agencies. Furthermore, there has been an increase in the number of other NGOs incorporating HIV and AIDS-related issues into the services they provide. These developments have taken place both within and beyond metropolitan authorities. However, health promotion and education programmes do not take place in a political vacuum and are largely controlled, in terms of their funding and feasibility, by priorities established elsewhere. In the context of HIV, this has meant that less mainstream yet vitally important health education programmes have at times been marginalised and undermined, since they may not conform to the 'norm'. Projects designed to work with men who have sex with men, those which explore the specific implications of HIV for black men and women, or for people with learning difficulties are examples (Evans, Sandberg and Watson, 1992).

HIV and AIDS have had a significant impact on the provision of services within all statutory and local authority organisations. They have created new demands in housing, social services support, primary and secondary health care, formal and non-formal education services—the list is endless. Yet it is probably local health promotion, given the current emphasis on prevention, that has been most acutely challenged by the advent of HIV and AIDS. There are now clear indicators about the sorts of health education strategies that are most effective and those which are less so. Most health educators now agree that large-scale media campaigns, videos and leaflets are not sufficient. At best, and in isolation, they are ineffectual but harmless; at worst, when coupled with the misinformation, myths and prejudiced notions perpetuated by the tabloid press, they can reinforce confusion, fear and prejudice. Mass health education campaigns in the mid-1980s promoted the idea that there were 'high-risk' groups and consequently generated a diehard disassociation from HIV and AIDS by those people who did not identify with being gay, an injecting drug user, a 'prostitute' or least of all 'promiscuous'. Health education messages bent on reinforcing moral codes are even less helpful, since they deny the diversity of individual and community attitudes towards, and expressions of, sexuality, and alienate large numbers of people who cannot identify with the message. Health promotion strategies which are based on the assumption that giving people information about health will lead to subsequent changes in lifestyle and the rejection of 'unhealthy' habits and behaviours are clearly highly inadequate in the face of HIV and AIDS. Exhortations to 'use a condom' have failed to address the complexities of negotiating safer sex, particularly for women, and of encouraging sustained changes in behaviour.

Yet in the 1990s HIV and AIDS health promotion in the UK still faces a number of problems in attempting to develop and institute the kind of health education which is most effective in relation to HIV and AIDS. Although statutory organisations are beginning to integrate HIV and AIDS education into their corporate strategies as and when the need arises, these moves continue to be mainly reactive instead of proactive. In some instances this is less of an issue for those undergoing training within a particular profession than it is for personnel who are established in post. Curriculum provision for HIV and AIDS has certainly been made within social work training, for example (CCETSW, 1992), and is being made, though often on an ad hoc basis (according to local authority policy), in other professional areas such as probation and environmental health.

However, there are still many people whose professional curricula have not addressed HIV and AIDS issues, or who qualified before relevant training programmes were established and who consequently have not been given opportunities to consider the potential impact of HIV on their work. With the plethora of new legislation affecting various areas of work, such as the Children Act, and the National Curriculum, it is easy to see why limited resources for in-service training have been earmarked for necessary guidance on these documents, and why HIV-related issues have been marginalised. Commitment is needed from the senior management of such organisations to identify clear links between HIV and other legislative developments and training priorities. In many instances it is possible to incorporate HIV and AIDS basic awareness into in-service training on, for example, the Children Act and children's rights, the National Curriculum, equal opportunities or child protection. At other times, depending on the context within which people are working, it is vital that separate and more substantial HIV and AIDS awareness training is made available to all personnel, and the pressures on managers to prioritise must not detract from this.

For preventive strategies to have any effect, a basic awareness level of good HIV and AIDS education must be made available across all sectors and through appropriate channels. *Learning About AIDS: Scientific and Social Issues* and *Learning About AIDS: Training Guidance and Exercises*, the participatory training resource which can be used with this book, have been designed to support such education by providing a comprehensive package of factual information and training guidance.

Opportunities to clarify medical and scientific knowledge of how the virus works and, above all, the chance to consider and review personal attitudes and beliefs in relation to HIV and AIDS are crucial. This constitutes the basic or 'homogeneous' level of education, examining common aspects of HIV and AIDS that affect us all. While it is essential that such issues be considered within an equal opportunities framework, this in itself is not enough to guarantee equal access to good education.

The reality is that societies are not homogeneous but comprise numerous situations where individuals may share things in common and have similar needs, but which are distinct from other situations. In the context of HIV and AIDS these needs may be determined by gender, sexuality, culture, class, religion, age, ethnicity, language, power, physical and mental abilities, employment, housing and any combination of the above. While it is vital to acknowledge that health education approaches informed by the 'high-risk group' theories of the mid-1980s are misguided and dangerous, it is important to acknowledge this differentiation of needs and its implications for providing good HIV and AIDS education. The potential for anyone promoting HIV and AIDS education lies in identifying those situations where people with common concerns choose to interact and which therefore provide opportunities for work with them. Once these have been identified, it is possible to employ principles of participation and empowerment in assessing needs, and in planning and implementing appropriate interventions that provide what people are looking for.

During the last decade or so HIV and AIDS education, often by trial and error, has highlighted a number of key principles which underlie good health promotion activities. First and foremost, it is almost impossible to devise good-quality health education interventions without establishing what the real training and learning needs are. A preliminary needs assessment which involves representatives from all who are to benefit from a programme or intervention is vital in determining its success. This serves a number of purposes. First, it is common sense to find out what is important to people by discussing their needs with them and ascertaining what will help them address those needs. Secondly, once a code of practice or way of working has been established, an ongoing needs assessment creates a dynamic situation where activities can be modified over time in accordance with changing needs. Thirdly, a needs assessment can establish criteria for evaluation and can be used to generate funding for further programme development. Fourthly, and most importantly, it can enable common and distinct interests to be established which inform practice in the sense of who will work most productively together on both individual and corporate levels. Finally, it will identify areas outside the competencies of those on any project team, and provide useful indicators concerning outside agencies that might offer support to address these needs.

Within the context of HIV and AIDS education, a needs assessment can raise the profile of HIV where this may not be recognised as a priority area. It will provide opportunities to draw links between identified needs and the importance of incorporating HIV-related issues within these. The links in question will vary according to the differing cultures of organisations and sectors, and may range from policy issues, such as equal opportunities and confidentiality, to risk minimisation, safer sex and sexuality education, or equal access to care provision. Indeed, ongoing needs assessment informed the development of this second edition of *Learning About AIDS: Scientific and Social Issues*, and enabled adaptations to be made in accordance with identified training needs.

For effective work to take place, HIV and AIDS health promotion must have participation as one of its basic tenets. In practice this must take place at every level, from initial policy development and needs assessment through to participatory learning styles in a workshop situation. At present, despite the separate involvement of statutory health, education, social services and local authority departments, there is still a distinct lack of communication between these sectors, and the benefits of intersectoral and multidisciplinary work are largely underestimated. A greater emphasis on participation and collaboration makes good economic sense: it is a means of sharing human and material resources, avoiding duplication of work and encouraging a coherent approach to good policy and practice.

This current dissected response to HIV and AIDS creates barriers to change on every level, yet there are numerous examples of effective collaboration on a micro level which, if adopted on a larger scale, would benefit not only HIV and AIDS programmes but health education provision as a whole. These are most commonly witnessed among voluntary sector and non-governmental organisations which, by the nature of their 'culture', appear to have a more flexible approach to working, making the obvious links between services where necessary and having greater success in providing education and support services. Body Positive groups, Positively Women, the Terrence Higgins Trust and numerous other non-AIDS-specific organisations offering advice and support for people with or concerned about HIV, people with AIDS, their partners, families, friends and carers, are just some of the responses there have been to the 'real' effects of HIV and AIDS. Such groups play a key role in health education and in training others to offer good-quality services.

Recent community care legislation in the UK is likely to give rise to new alliances between the voluntary sector and local authorities, with the latter—the purchasers—commissioning services from the former, the providers. Yet there is a danger that such forced participation could reap more difficulties than benefits. It is vital in the context of AIDS that planners are aware of this, and that mechanisms are put in place so that potential difficulties in such alliances can be overcome. Statutory organisations may need to undergo some fundamental changes in their approaches, developing some of that same flexibility presently attributed to the voluntary sector. It will then be possible for workable partnerships between the voluntary and local authority sectors to be created, based on fair contracts which allow the autonomy and independence of voluntary organisations to be maintained.

On a planning level, participation should involve representatives from all relevant parties, above all from those whom a proposed intervention is designed to benefit. Needs and concerns cannot be assumed, and it is not possible to ascertain why previous initiatives have failed to reach their goals without entering into dialogue. If people have a chance to determine the nature of programmes for their own good, then they will have a sense of ownership and, most importantly, control over them. Such an approach is likely to be both beneficial and cost effective.

In terms of creating learning environments conducive to open discussion, participatory approaches have a lot to offer. Probably the most important advantage of participatory learning over other forms of education is the opportunities it creates to examine not only 'facts' but attitudes, beliefs and values in relation to all the issues that HIV and AIDS encompass: sex, sexuality, drug use, power structures, prejudice, homophobia, racism, discrimination etc. This enables participants to engage themselves on a level where they can remove their professional 'hats' and consider the effects of their personal attitudes and beliefs on their actions in and out of work. For example, it is unreasonable for a personal and social education tutor in school to offer young people guidance on safer sex and sexuality if he or she has never had an opportunity to reflect on his or her own feelings about these issues. Similarly, until care providers have had opportunities to think about how homophobic or moralising attitudes and values affect their relationship with people on the 'receiving end' of care, barriers in communication will persist.

Participatory learning, when handled well, allows information to be shared and not given, fears and myths to be dispelled and not hidden, people and their ideas to be valued and not talked down to and, above all, the chance for personal reflection and growth. The classic teacher–pupil approach to learning is replaced by the facilitator–participant style, where individuals and groups retain control and responsibility over their own learning. The facilitator's role within this process is a very special one and requires careful preparation.[1]

HIV and AIDS, more than any other health and social issues, have brought into the open discriminatory attitudes and practices which otherwise might have remained more covert and in some ways perhaps more difficult to confront and challenge. The relatively short history of AIDS and HIV has been riddled with homophobia and heterosexism, racism and judgementalism against those who appear not to conform. These prejudices still prevail, despite the shift emphasising the potential of HIV and AIDS to affect everybody. Yet the recent marginalisation of work

---

[1] The training guidance section included in the *Learning About AIDS* package is designed to offer support to those assuming a facilitation role; it is recommended for those who seek further assistance.

with gay and bisexual men, for example, and the lack of funds to validate this work, are indicators of attitudes commonly held by those in positions of authority and financial power (King, Rooney and Scott, 1992). So long as these standpoints pervade decision-making bodies, society as a whole will continue to accept discriminatory practices as the norm. Those responsible for devising HIV and AIDS health promotion strategies must consider how to address these attitudes at every level.

Creating learning environments where such prejudice and its impact are brought into question has far greater importance in the longer term than 'ironing' out minutiae in factual information. Further, health promoters and educators are often in positions where they can undertake work with the senior management and power brokers of organisations. It is in situations such as these that existing policies on equal access to good-quality health education, care and support services, as well as policies in relation to employment practice, housing and any other pertinent services, can be brought into question. HIV has created opportunities to distinguish reality from rhetoric where equity and antidiscrimination are concerned; and HIV and AIDS health promoters are often well placed to raise concerns about current practice.

This discussion has highlighted how much HIV and AIDS health promotion activity has had to be reviewed and adapted in accordance with its lack of success, or in response to changing needs and priorities. This inevitably underlines the importance of monitoring and evaluation in assessing both the impact of programmes and the personal effectiveness of those directly involved. Despite the understandable fears and reservations that are often expressed about evaluation, it is important to recognise that without it there can be neither progress nor the opportunity to take credit for success or learn from mistakes. Probably the most important incentive for evaluation is the guarantee of further funding for projects by proving that existing activities (or modified versions of them) represent money well spent.

Evaluation is no longer the domain of outside experts using complex scientific tools. While there may be some call for external evaluation, it is more likely, for economic reasons more than anything else, that health educators will be expected to devise evaluation tools for their own work. The resolution of issues about who should be involved in this process, when it should take place and how it should be planned and managed can take time and energy. The Health Education Authority's HIV/AIDS Local Evaluation Support Initiative was established to address concerns about effective evaluation specifically in the context of HIV and AIDS health promotion activities. We recommend some of the publications from this project as an initial reference point for anyone undertaking work in this area (e.g. Aggleton, Moody and Young, 1992; Aggleton, Young, Moody, Kapila and Pye, 1992).

It is within the context described above that subsequent chapters discuss a range of issues likely to be of importance in HIV and AIDS health promotion. Chapter 2 illustrates that there now exists a substantial body of knowledge about HIV and its effects. Besides confirming former evidence relating to the routes of transmission of HIV and its effects on the immune system, recent research is providing clearer indicators for the management and prophylactic treatment of HIV-related conditions. It is vital for health educators to develop a good working knowledge of HIV and AIDS and to keep in touch with new developments so that they can work effectively with groups and be able to convey factual information which is both useful and relevant to their needs. This book includes a basic description of the immune system and information on the different ways in which HIV disease may manifest itself in women, men and children.

Surveys of what people actually want to know about HIV and AIDS have revealed changes over recent years, reflecting the realisation that these conditions are affecting all of us and that preventive strategies are only one part of the picture. There have been repeated requests for more accessible information relating to available therapy, treatment and trials for HIV-related conditions. These are discussed in Chapter 3, which acknowledges current debate about orthodox treatments and alternative and complementary therapies. It also considers the politics of drug treatment trials, questions about equal opportunity for participation in these, and the ethics involved.

A statistical update on the prevalence and distribution of HIV infection and AIDS is invariably a learning priority. Chapter 4 explores the difficulties in establishing accurate data on the pattern or the extent of spread (the epidemiology) of HIV and AIDS on a local, national, continental and global scale. The dangers of overreliance on existing statistical data, without corroboration from more qualitative information, will be considered. In relation to existing data on the epidemic, issues about HIV antibody and antigen testing are discussed, as are the social and economic disincentives to testing. In the absence of any legislation to protect fundamental rights of HIV antibody-positive people to housing, employment, insurance and other basic human rights, and while even those who test negative are discriminated against, it is unlikely that a clearer epidemiological picture for HIV and AIDS will emerge.

Of course, the provision of relevant and up-to-date health information does not in itself constitute health education. In fact, studies of how much people actually know about HIV, especially those carried out among young people, consistently reveal high levels of knowledge and awareness. Evidently this 'knowing' is not enough, and unfortunately there is no direct link between this and attitude and behaviour change. This is true of any type of health promotion, but HIV and AIDS are fraught with sensitivities since they touch on areas of people's lives that many may find difficult to address, above all sex, sexuality and drug use. Chapter 5 examines issues to do with promoting sexual health in the light of HIV and AIDS from a more holistic viewpoint than the nuts and bolts of safer sex. Factors that determine whether or not safer sex is introduced into a relationship, such as assertiveness, self-esteem, negotiation and communications skills, language and culture, are discussed, as are the implications for health promotion activities.

Chapter 6 investigates the links between drug use and the risk of HIV infection. It illustrates how laws have determined some drugs illicit and others licit. Although the direct link between HIV and injected drug use, where 'works' are shared, is commonly made, there is limited recognition of the possible links between HIV infection and the use of alcohol or psychoactive drugs which can mar judgement when making choices about minimising the risks of HIV transmission and/or other sexually transmitted diseases (STDs). Emphasis is placed on the need to adopt a non-judgemental and non-discriminatory stance when working with people who use currently illicit drugs. A clear argument is advanced for the establishment of collaborative and multidisciplinary approaches which develop HIV-related work with drug programmes in both the voluntary and statutory sectors. These would allow the interrelationships of sexual health, drugs (in their broadest sense) and harm minimisation to be more fully appreciated, and would help to avoid the all-too-common situation in which drug-related issues are considered in isolation.

Chapter 7 highlights the benefits and importance of successful intersectoral work for people living with HIV and AIDS. It shows how a lack of collaboration and coordination in the past has resulted in inadequate and even harmful responses towards those seeking help and support. Attention is drawn to some of the personal, organisational and political barriers to thinking constructively about HIV and AIDS and, in particular, to the role of health educators and promoters in heightening public awareness so that HIV disease is recognised for what it is, a major threat to health and wellbeing.

2

HIV and AIDS

Edward King   Peter Scott   Peter Aggleton

AIDS is a diagnosis given when a person has a certain set of symptoms which have resulted from damage to the human immune system caused by a virus known as HIV (the human immunodeficiency virus). It is important to have a basic knowledge both of the immune system and of viruses in order to understand what the disease is and how it might be treated.

THE HUMAN IMMUNE SYSTEM

The body's immune system protects us from harmful organisms such as viruses, bacteria or fungi. However, in some people the immune system does not function properly. This may be due to a hereditary malfunction, deliberate medical suppression of the immune system (for example, to prevent rejection of transplanted organs), or to HIV infection. If the immune system is impaired, opportunistic infections—so called because they are caused by organisms which are normally not harmful but which 'take the opportunity' to cause disease because damage to the immune system has left the body vulnerable—may occur. Opportunistic infections are often caused by common organisms, which are present in many people but which go unnoticed and are unable to cause harm because the normally functioning immune system keeps them suppressed. Where there is damage to the immune system (often referred to as immunosuppression or immunodeficiency) these infections are able to cause illness which can be life-threatening.

The structure of the immune system

The immune system is a term used to describe the mechanisms through which the body protects itself from organisms which, unchecked, may cause disease (*pathogens* or *pathogenic organisms*). In addition to physical barriers such as the skin and mucous membranes, which protect us against pathogenic organisms, specialised cells in our bloodstream inactivate pathogenic micro-organisms such as bacteria and viruses.

Within the body there are many specialised immune system cells which move through the bloodstream and lymphatic system to get to infected or wounded tissue. The majority of these cells only live for days or weeks. New cells are constantly produced from parent cells in the bone marrow.

Non-specific immunity (phagocytes)

An important type of cell in the immune system are the white blood cells called phagocytes, which specialise in recognising and destroying micro-organisms, such as bacteria, by secreting toxins. There are two types of phagocytes: macrophages and the granulocytes. Granulocytes are probably not affected by HIV (Figure 2.1). Macrophages, however, are infected by HIV and this is particularly important since, when healthy, they are able to ingest large pathogenic organisms and are also capable of destroying cancerous cells. However, in HIV disease macrophages may in fact constitute a reservoir of the virus because they can survive for months or years and move freely around the body.

Specific immunity (lymphocytes)

More complex animals, including human beings, have developed a second large class of immune cells: the lymphocytes. These are able to recognise and selectively target a given virus or bacterium. The human body contains billions of lymphocytes, disseminated throughout the blood, the spleen, the lymph nodes and other specialist organs such as the appendix, the tonsils and the adenoids.

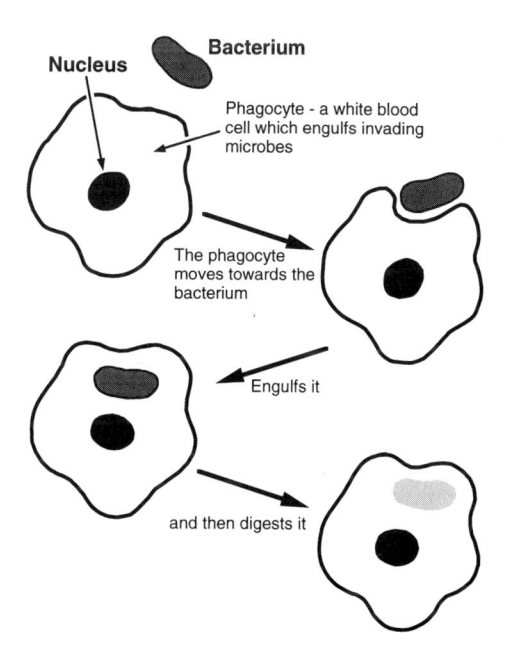

Figure 2.1 A phagocyte engulfing a bacterium.

Lymphocytes are produced by groups of identical cells, or clones, which are all descended from the same parent cell. Each lymphocyte clone is 'programmed' to recognise a particular pathogenic agent or, to be more precise, a fragment (or antigen) from that pathogen. This antigen may be, for example, a viral protein, a molecule in the bacterial cell wall or a bacterial toxin. It is estimated that about 10 million different lymphocytes are circulating in the blood, potentially ready to respond to 10 million different pathogens. When infection occurs, cells such as macrophages identify pathogenic organisms, absorb them and then present recognisable fragments of these organisms to lymphocytes, which are then activated and search for the organisms throughout the body in order to destroy them.

Humoral immunity One large subset of lymphocytes, the B lymphocytes, circulates constantly in the blood and lymph systems and plays a central role in the body's immune system.

B cells emit antibodies to attack pathogens. Each B lymphocyte is programmed to recognise a particular antigen and to secrete antibodies capable of targeting it.

Each type of antibody is shaped so that it can attach itself to a particular shape of antigen (in a mirror image of the way the virus attaches itself to a cell wall). This, in itself, may prevent the virus binding to a cell by blocking its binding mechanism. Additionally, the attachment of the antibodies brings about the recognition and digestion of the antigen by phagocytes (Figure 2.2). Antibodies can also deal with a virus that is circulating freely in the bloodstream. However, in most viral infections the majority of the virus is hidden away within host cells. The antibody-based system cannot fight the virus here and another system (the cell-mediated system) is needed to destroy the virus by identifying and destroying the body's own infected cells.

Cell-mediated immunity There is a further subset of lymphocytes called T cells. T cells are themselves divided into different types: cytotoxic T cells (also known as CD8 cells), which are able to move through body tissues, recognise cells which have been

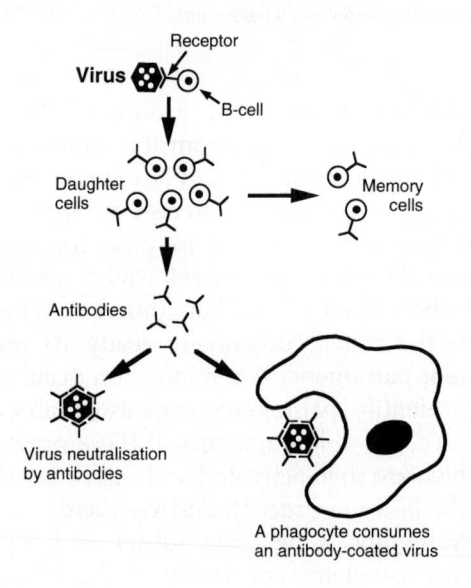

Figure 2.2 Processes involving B cells.

infected by viruses or bacteria, adhere to them and destroy them, and helper T cells (also known as CD4 cells or T4 cells), which form the majority of the total number of T cells and are identified by a surface molecule or marker called CD4. These cells actually set the immune response in motion by activating B cells which secrete antibodies. They also release chemical stimulators which activate cytotoxic cells and the macrophages.

In our lifetime we all encounter a number of pathogens to which we develop immunity. Memory cells, which can be B cells or T cells, remember specific antigens so that any subsequent infection can be dealt with much more quickly by simply reactivating the memories represented within these cells.

VACCINES

Vaccines work by exploiting the memory mechanism of the immune system. A vaccine is basically one or more parts of a virus which have been made chemically harmless. When this is introduced into the body, the same range of immune responses develops against the harmless fragments as would develop against the whole pathogen. As a result, if there is a subsequent exposure to the whole virus, the memory cells of the immune system are already equipped with the pattern of its antigens and so can produce a massive response much more quickly. Boosters work by refreshing this cellular memory from time to time.

WHAT IS HIV?

It is almost universally acknowledged that HIV is the virus whose harmful effects on the immune system can lead to AIDS. This section explains the lifecycle of viruses in general, and of HIV in particular. However, a few writers and commentators have suggested that HIV is not the cause of AIDS. This view is discussed later in this chapter.

Introduction to viruses

Viruses are the simplest form of life. They are microscopically

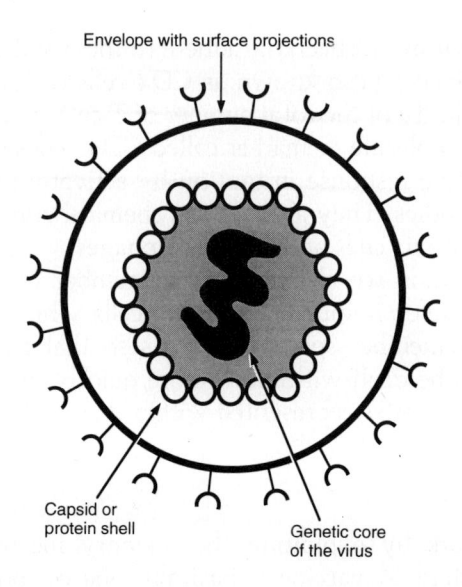

Figure 2.3 The main features of a virus.

small and made up of a number of different parts. Like cells, viruses have an outer coat made of a mixture of fats, sugars and proteins which contains genetic material and enzymes. A virus consists of three main parts (Figure 2.3):

- the viral 'coat' or envelope, made up of proteins and complex sugars;
- the core proteins and enzymes which are used in the production of a new virus;
- the genetic material in the form of deoxyribonucleic acid (DNA) or ribonucleic acid (RNA), which determines how the virus will reproduce itself.

To keep a description of viruses simple, it is common to use phrases such as: 'the virus aims to ...' or 'the virus has a way of ...'. It is important to bear in mind, however, that this is only a convenient shorthand. The way viruses work is not the result of planning, desire or thinking. Their actions develop through evolution: genetic mutation and natural selection.

From a biological viewpoint the sole aim of any virus (like any other form of life) is to reproduce its genetic message. However, unlike most other forms of life, a virus cannot grow independently but can only reproduce itself inside the cells of other living organisms. Although a virus can survive outside its host, it can only do so in a dormant (or resting) state. It cannot grow or reproduce outside its host, because it is a simple form of life that lacks all the complex characteristics of more highly developed cells.

Each different species (or type) of virus can infect particular host species. Although some viruses can infect different species, most are specific to one particular host species. This explains why viral diseases common to some animals are not common to others.

Each virus has a specific way of getting inside the body of its host: it may be carried in blood, in sexual fluids, through drinking water, in contaminated food or in an aerosol of tiny droplets produced by sneezing. Although viruses can mutate or alter by changing the shape or structure of their outer coat and thus becoming more or less infectious, it is very, very unlikely for a virus to mutate in such a manner as to change the way it infects its hosts. For instance, common cold viruses are transmitted through sneezing, whereas HIV is transmitted through blood and sexual fluids.

Once inside the body of the host, the virus 'binds' on to the wall of a host cell. It can do this because the coat of the virus has proteins which are shaped to fit and lock onto particular proteins on the cell wall. This is often described as similar to the way in which a particular key fits a particular lock.

Once the virus has locked on to the host cell, it can start to enter the cell. Fats in the surface of the virus start to mix with fats on the surface of the cell; the surfaces of both become fused, and the inner contents of the virus—genetic material and enzymes— enter the cell. Inside the cell the virus inserts (or integrates) the viral genetic material (called the provirus) into the nucleus of the host cell. Once there, the provirus cannot be removed during the lifetime of the cell.

The virus may then remain 'dormant' for a period before it is 'activated'. This activation may occur almost immediately or after many years, depending on the nature of the virus and its host. In addition, the virus in only some cells may become activated in this way. When the infected cell is activated and needs to read its own genetic message (perhaps in order to reproduce or replace itself), the genetic message of the provirus is also read and can override the cell's own message. The viral DNA directs enzymes belonging to the host cell to produce the raw materials for making a new virus, which can then go on to infect new cells.

Because viruses operate by incorporating their own genetic material alongside the genetic material of the host cells, they pose special problems for medicine, as it is unlikely that a virus can be eradicated without also destroying the cells that contain it. Equally, it may be difficult to reach a dormant virus that is hidden inactively within apparently normal host cells. Because the virus uses the cell's own mechanisms to produce new virus, it can be difficult to produce drugs that attack the lifecycle of the virus without also doing serious damage to the human cells as well. This is why, in general, antiviral drugs are harder to develop than drugs to deal with bacterial or fungal infections.

Retroviruses

HIV is a member of a family of viruses called retroviruses. Science has only a limited experience of these: the first human retrovirus, HTLV-1 (human T-lymphotropic virus type 1), was only isolated as recently as 1980. Retroviruses are different from other viruses: their genetic message is stored in a chemical molecule called RNA (ribonucleic acid). Humans (and most other forms of life including other viruses) have their genetic message stored in a different molecule, called DNA (deoxyribonucleic acid).

Because the genetic message of retroviruses is contained in RNA, there is an extra step in their lifecycle. Most viruses simply incorporate their existing DNA into the DNA in the nucleus of the host cell. In retroviruses, including HIV, the information flow of the genetic message goes in the reverse direction. Retroviruses convert their RNA into DNA first, and then incorporate this viral DNA into the host cell's own DNA. This is important for two reasons: on the one hand it makes the retrovirus harder to eradicate, and on the other hand it provides a point of attack specific to the lifecycle of this group of viruses, namely the enzyme called reverse transcriptase which converts viral RNA into viral DNA (Gallo, 1991).

HIV AND THE IMMUNE SYSTEM

HIV attacks and infects the very cells of the immune system that exist to fight infection. A molecule on the outside of HIV, called gp120, can bind tightly on to a molecule called CD4 in the cell wall of the helper T lymphocytes that are so important in cell-mediated immunity (Figures 2.4 and 2.5). These T cells are the main kind of cell which is depleted from the body in the course of HIV disease. There are also CD4 receptors on a range of other cells, including macrophages, some B cells and some brain cells. There are other ways that HIV can enter cells, but the binding of

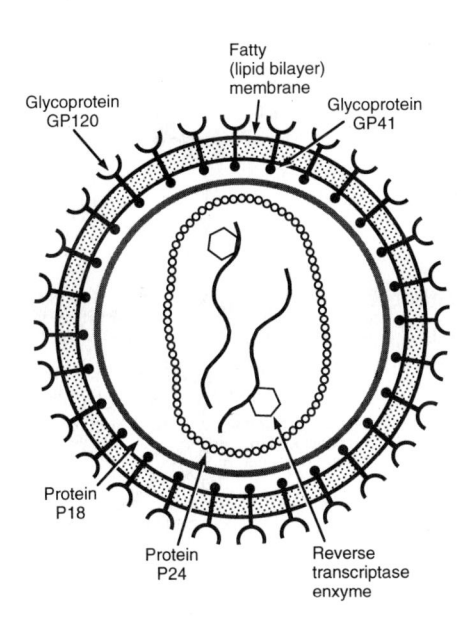

Figure 2.4 The structure of HIV.

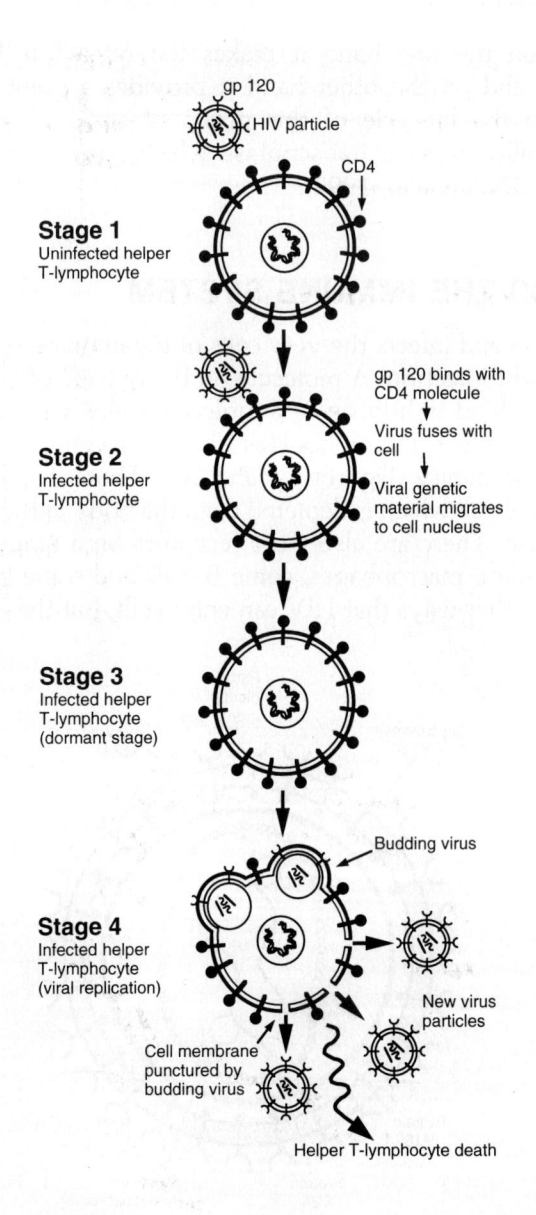

Figure 2.5 The lifecycle of HIV.

gp120 to CD4 is the main way in which it infects the most important cells: CD4 lymphocytes and macrophages.

After HIV has attached itself to the CD4 receptor, it injects its core into the cell. This allows the viral RNA and enzymes to mingle with the contents of the human cell. Then, as described earlier, viral RNA is converted into viral DNA. Once HIV has inserted its genetic message, it is there for the lifetime of the cell and can be eliminated only if the cell is killed. Because the virus can remain in a dormant state for a considerable time period (thought to be up to 12 years), a person who has become infected may remain asymptomatic—that is, healthy and without any symptoms of diseases related to HIV—for long periods. Others may experience skin rashes, fevers, night sweats, swollen glands or diarrhoea. However, these are not reliable indicators of HIV infection and can be symptoms of a number of other common infections and conditions, including stress. For this reason, the majority of people who have HIV infection are not aware of it. Nevertheless, during the period of dormancy, it is possible to pass HIV on, not just to other cells in the body but to other people through infected cells in the blood and in sexual fluids (see Chapter 4). The HIV-infected cell can become activated by a number of factors: certain other infections are most likely to cause this. Once an HIV-infected cell has been activated, the viral DNA is converted to viral RNA which uses enzymes to make viral proteins. The various viral components migrate to the surface of the cell as they are formed, and are assembled there. These new viruses are emitted out of the cell wall and go on to infect other cells. It is likely that the infected cell is killed in the final process of the virus being emitted and moving on to infect other cells.

HOW HIV CAUSES DISEASE

The way in which a particular disease is caused is known as pathogenesis. Despite the extensive research into AIDS over the last 10 years, surprisingly little is known about the precise mechanisms by which HIV can result in AIDS. It should be stressed that the incomplete nature of our knowledge about the pathogenesis of AIDS does not mean that HIV is not the cause of

AIDS. What is unclear is what happens between the moment of infection with HIV and the later onset of AIDS—and why the time between these events is so variable from person to person. We know that HIV does cause AIDS somehow, and with the renewed attention given to this question, some light is beginning to be shed on the mechanisms involved.

Theories of pathogenesis

Early studies of people with AIDS revealed that CD4 T cell counts were significantly lowered. When HIV was identified and found to infect cells via the CD4 receptor, it was initially assumed that HIV was simply infecting CD4 cells and killing them—the theory of direct cytopathicity. This theory became—at least temporarily—less acceptable when it became clear that only relatively few CD4 cells in the blood of people with HIV are actually infected with the virus. Furthermore, very few of the infected cells contain a virus that is active: in most of them the virus is integrated into the cells' DNA in a stage of complete dormancy.

However, recent technological advances have enabled researchers to observe that HIV is present in the blood at levels up to ten times higher than could previously be detected (Pantaleo et al, 1993), but researchers still disagree on whether enough cells are infected for the direct cytopathicity theory to be a full explanation of CD4 cell loss. Other theories have been proposed suggesting that HIV can indirectly cause uninfected immune system cells to be destroyed or to stop functioning normally. This may be by:

- forming syncytia—a few infected CD4 T cells may gather uninfected T cells around them, forming a clump of cells called a syncytium. All the cells of the syncytium then die, whether they are HIV-infected or not;
- releasing the viral protein gp120 into the bloodstream. This may stick to CD4 cells, stopping them from functioning properly, or may fool the immune system into thinking that the cells are infected with HIV and destroying them;

- programming immune cells to commit suicide (a process called apoptosis, or programmed cell death) when they are activated, regardless of whether they are actually infected with HIV;
- causing other disturbances in the immune system which mislead it into attacking its own cells. This phenomenon is known as autoimmunity;
- disrupting the body's system of chemical messengers (called cytokines).

Other theories highlight the fact that HIV can infect or disregulate other important cells of the body, including immune system sentinels in the skin and mucous membranes (known as dendritic cells), the lymph nodes and the cytotoxic CD8 cells. Some people may also be more vulnerable to HIV than others, depending on their individual genetic make-up. HIV may be able to evade the immune system by its frequent mutations, and different strains of the virus may be much more harmful than others. This field of research is still very active (Levy, 1993).

DISEASE PROGRESSION AND COFACTORS

The longer a person has been infected with HIV, the more likely it is that their immune system will be impaired and they will be vulnerable to opportunistic infections. We do not know exactly why one person with HIV infection develops AIDS and another does not. As with most infectious diseases, one factor may be individual genetic heredity. Another factor may be age: older people and babies tend to experience faster disease progression than young adults.

In addition, various avoidable cofactors have been suggested, because they are directly immunosuppressive (such as some recreational drugs), because they may stimulate HIV to do further damage (such as certain herpes viruses and other sexually transmitted diseases), or because they would make the impact of an opportunistic infection more severe. Theories about cofactors have come and gone. For example, it used to be thought that women with HIV risked faster disease progression if they became pregnant. This has been demonstrated not to be the case.

The existence of cofactors to HIV does not mean that the cofactors cause AIDS on their own, in the absence of HIV. Nor does it mean that HIV may not cause AIDS on its own, in the absence of cofactors.

Does disease progression differ between social groups?

Some studies have appeared to show that HIV disease progresses faster in certain population groups than others. For example, as noted above, age does appear to have a significant effect on individual prognosis, and early research studies suggested that women with HIV progressed to AIDS more rapidly than men. However, more detailed research strongly suggests that any such effect is due to poorer or later access to medical diagnosis and treatment, rather than to any important biological differences in the effects of HIV within the male and female bodies.

Tests for disease progression

Laboratory tests can be used to monitor disease progression in people infected with HIV. As such, they provide back-up information to clinical examinations by a doctor. However, it is important to understand that there is genuine 'good faith' disagreement between different doctors about what significance to attach to laboratory markers when treating and caring for an individual. In the UK the routine tests performed are:

- a lymphocyte subset analysis which counts the number of CD4 cells in a cubic millimetre of blood (usually called the CD4 cell count);
- sometimes a test for the HIV core protein p24 antigen, or antibodies produced by the body against this protein.

Other laboratory measures, such as β_2-microglobulin and neopterin tests, tend not to be used routinely, but often just during clinical trials of HIV treatments. More recent developments include quantitative tests which can measure the amount of virus itself in a blood or tissue sample.

HOW DO WE KNOW THAT HIV IS THE CAUSE?

Our understanding of HIV and AIDS is new and limited. Consequently, there is a range of unresolved issues which can be presented together as a challenge to the theory that HIV is the cause of AIDS. For example, the apparently different rates of progression in different individuals and different populations can lead to the belief that there cannot be a single underlying cause. The fact that most, if not all, of the opportunistic infections to which people with HIV are vulnerable can also affect people uninfected with HIV (for example, transplant recipients) can lead to at least two mistaken assumptions: that AIDS is not new, and that some people uninfected with HIV but who have certain opportunistic conditions, such as Kaposi's sarcoma (KS), which is a form of skin cancer, actually have AIDS.

The changing definition of AIDS may also lead to confusion. AIDS is not defined by the presence of HIV alone: its definition is based upon a range of disorders that comprise a syndrome. HIV has to be present alongside these other disorders for a case of AIDS to be diagnosed.

In some countries, the continuing (though not exclusive) concentration of AIDS in groups such as gay men and injecting drug users where 'lifestyle' characteristics can be casually assumed or identified may be misinterpreted to argue that it is aspects of that lifestyle, rather than an infectious agent, which is responsible for the epidemic.

However, scientific evidence from thousands of studies around the world overwhelmingly confirms that HIV plays a central role in the AIDS epidemic. We know a great deal about HIV, although there are some gaps in our understanding of exactly how it works at a cellular level to produce varying degrees of damage to the immune system in different people over time. We know that the cause of AIDS has to be a transmissible agent, and that HIV is the only candidate that fits all the affected groups in the epidemic. As our understanding of AIDS has improved, the theory that HIV is not the cause of AIDS has become weaker (Weiss, 1993).

WHAT IS AIDS?

It is important to be clear that AIDS is not a single disease but a syndrome made up of many possible diseases. Therefore, people can experience the course of HIV disease and AIDS in many different ways, and the prognosis cannot be the same for any two individuals.

Opportunistic conditions

A person with HIV is diagnosed as having AIDS if they develop certain specific opportunistic infections or tumours. The opportunistic infections which are considered to be AIDS-defining are specifically listed in the official definition of AIDS drawn up by the Centers for Disease Control (CDC) in the USA (CDC, 1992). They include:

- protozoal infections such as *Toxoplasma gondii*, *Cryptosporidium* and *Isospora belli*;
- bacterial infections such as *Mycobacterium tuberculosis* (TB) and *Mycobacterium avium intracellulare* (MAI);
- fungal infections such as *Pneumocystis carinii* (PCP, previously believed to be a protozoan), *Candida albicans* and *Cryptococcus neoformans*;
- viral infections such as cytomegalovirus (CMV), herpes simplex (HSV) and zoster (HZV or VZV), and human papilloma virus (HPV).

CDC definitions of stages of HIV infection

The CDC case definitions for AIDS have evolved over time as the shape of the epidemic has changed. The pressures for changes in the definitions come from epidemiologists and clinical trial organisers, as well as officials involved in budgeting and mobilising health care and AIDS treatment activists. Although each definition may represent a refinement, they tend to include more individuals, rather than fewer, and so people suddenly find that overnight they are being categorised as having AIDS, with no real change in their physical status.

As it became obvious that children infected with HIV had a different spectrum of problems, and because of the difficulty of diagnosing HIV infection in children under 15 months old, special paediatric diagnostic criteria were introduced.

Other definitions

The CDC definitions above take into account only the experience in the USA, and may be less useful in the UK and Europe, where some of the AIDS-defining diagnoses are very rare because of the differences in environmental pathogens. They are certainly almost useless in Africa and other less developed areas, where the marked differences in environment result in a different clinical picture, and where the absence of high-technology laboratories means that some infections (e.g. CMV, MAI) would be very difficult to diagnose.

To try to redress these issues, the World Health Organization has developed special definitions for adults and children in Africa. According to these, AIDS in an adult is defined by the existence of at least two listed 'major signs', such as dramatic weight loss, diarrhoea or fever, and one 'minor sign' such as candida, cough, rash or swollen lymph nodes, in the absence of other known causes of immunosuppression such as cancer or malnutrition. The diagnoses of Kaposi's sarcoma and cryptococcal meningitis are sufficient in themselves for a diagnosis of AIDS. In children, two major and two minor signs must be present. A positive HIV test is not a prerequisite.

The WHO criteria for both children and adults have, however, been criticised as being too insensitive (they do not pick up all the cases of AIDS) and too non-specific (they mistakenly diagnose some people as having AIDS).

Debates about the definition

In reality, not all AIDS-defining disorders have the same prognosis or outlook. For example, a gay man with a single lesion of Kaposi's sarcoma has AIDS, but has a better outlook than a gay man with PCP, another common AIDS-defining disorder. Age, race, gender and lifestyle factors can also mean that people who have the same rigidly defined HIV illnesses may have very different prospects. Nevertheless, rigid definitions can be very useful in some circumstances. For example, in clinical and epidemiological studies, when large populations of people are being observed, it is essential to have well defined 'endpoints' as points of comparison. This is the only way that scientific principles can be adhered to and the studies can reach firm, reliable conclusions. It is also appropriate that these definitions change from time to time, as the epidemic evolves and we find out more.

Women's concerns

There has been some concern that the current definition was based on the opportunistic conditions seen particularly in gay men, and that it therefore omits important conditions which are specific to women. These might include cervical cancer (caused by human papilloma virus, HPV) and pelvic inflammatory disease (PID).

It is argued that HIV-related illnesses in women are not being properly diagnosed and treated, and that women are being denied access to services and benefits which are available to people who have been diagnosed with AIDS. There has therefore been pressure for the definition of AIDS to be revised to include women-specific opportunistic infections and tumours. However, there has been some dispute over the merits of extending the definition, as conditions such as HPV and PID are also not uncommon causes of morbidity among sexually active women who are not infected with HIV.

More recently, the CDC has changed its definition entirely, so that any person with HIV who has a CD4 count less than 200 is said to have AIDS, regardless of symptoms or opportunistic conditions. However, this definition has also been heavily criticised because it is based upon laboratory tests rather than clinical diagnoses. In European countries the AIDS definition remains based on the diagnosis of specific conditions, and does not include having a CD4 count less than 200.

HIV disease as a spectrum

Definitions of HIV and AIDS as they have evolved have come to suggest that HIV infection is an inevitable, one-way process. In other words, they imply that everyone with HIV will initially be well, then they will have abnormal tests a little while before they become mildly ill, and finally there will be a severe terminal illness. Although this has indeed been the pattern for many people, others have had very different experiences. For example, some people can contract infections that would be diagnostic of AIDS and then become healthy again for a long while. This may be because their immune systems were damaged by a combination of HIV and another, temporary cofactor which went away (for example, stress or another infection).

Moreover, the development of new and improved treatments for both the underlying HIV infection and the opportunistic infections has significantly altered the natural history of HIV and AIDS. Early estimates of the proportion of people with HIV who will go on to develop AIDS were based partly on the experience of the epidemic in the years before drugs such as AZT (see Chapter 3) became widely available. As new drugs against HIV and opportunistic infections gradually become available, these too may have an impact on estimates of the average prognosis of people with HIV.

In the earlier years of the epidemic the term ARC (AIDS-related complex) was widely used to describe the health of people with relatively minor HIV-related symptoms or infections which were not considered to be AIDS-defining. More recently, however, ARC and also, to a lesser extent, AIDS, have been recognised as unsatisfactory terms, limited by historical accident. Many doctors now prefer to think of HIV disease or HIV infection and disease. This approach sees HIV and the symptoms and opportunistic infections that can result from HIV infection as a spectrum of problems, without well defined phases. People with HIV disease may have dramatically different experiences of the condition, including being entirely asymptomatic, occasionally having symptoms of varying severity but also long periods of good health, and being quite sick.

3

Treatment and therapy

Edward King   Peter Scott

HIV/AIDS medicine is a very young specialty, and the human immunodeficiency virus (HIV) behaves in a very complex way. The successful development of drugs against HIV requires an understanding of the finely balanced and intricate interactions between the virus and the human body. Although major discoveries and new insights can be made, the task is basically a slow, gradual investigation. Any new drug must be understood as a small step along this long-term path. It may offer real immediate benefits, or it may be beset by side effects. Either way it is likely to be unclear at the outset of any treatment or trial what that drug will achieve in the long run.

SOME PROVISOS

Expectations are easily raised, especially by the mass media. The hype surrounding promising drugs should always be set against the cautious evaluation that any researcher or doctor will give. There are four main ways in which the process of developing new treatments can go wrong or be misunderstood; these are discussed in the following paragraphs.

Laboratory studies and human studies

Test tube studies, also known as in vitro (meaning 'in glass') studies, are used to see whether drugs have effects against HIV growing in human cells kept alive outside the human body. Many antiretroviral drugs have been tested in vitro but have not been found to be helpful in vivo (in the human body). Over the past 10 years there have been frequent press reports of promising drugs which have been effective against HIV in vitro but have not proved useful in practice.

Poorly conducted studies

Not only can laboratory studies give misleading impressions about the promise of candidate drugs; so, too, can human studies or clinical trials. This has been a particular problem in HIV/AIDS research. The drug ribavirin, for example, was first shown to be effective in vitro in 1984. Within a year clinical trials were under way. This study was rapidly completed and the results were publicised at the International AIDS Conference in 1987. The study focused on people with asymptomatic HIV infection and seemed to show that the control group receiving a placebo was nine times more likely to develop AIDS than the group receiving ribavirin. But the rate at which the placebo group was becoming sick was surprisingly high—18% over 7 months. When the data from the trial were studied more closely, it became apparent that members of the placebo group had had much lower CD4 counts at the beginning of the study: in this situation almost any drug would have falsely been shown to be effective.

As a result of this trial, several countries licensed ribavirin for use in HIV infection. However, the trial was heavily criticised by the FDA (the drug licensing authority in the USA). For a while many people with HIV felt that some kind of conspiracy had taken place, and consequently ribavirin became a widely used, secretly imported, underground drug. Several studies since then seem to have shown that ribavirin on its own does not have any clear benefits, and enthusiasm has waned considerably.

Mass media misunderstanding and hype

Each new drug that shows even a small beneficial effect tends to be given immense media publicity. Similarly, reports in the mass media tend to cause confusion by presenting early laboratory advances in, say, vaccine development as if they were breakthroughs in clinical treatment.

The hyping of particular drugs does not happen only in the mass media. It is understandable that, given a limited number of licensed antiviral drugs, there will always be pressure within community and activist groups to emphasise the more hopeful aspects of a new and experimental drug rather than its possible drawbacks.

The pace and structure of the drug development system

There is no international coordination of drug development to maximise the effectiveness of available resources in finding the most effective treatments as quickly as possible. The rivalries of individual investigators and of pharmaceutical companies can delay the process of a drug's development, no matter how promising it may appear on the shelf. A new kind of activism has developed in response to the AIDS epidemic which seeks to address key issues such as the pace of research, the direction of the enquiry, the involvement of community groups and the ethics and efficacy of trial design (Arno and Feiden, 1992; Kramer, 1990).

CAUTIOUS OPTIMISM

Despite these provisos, there are grounds for cautious optimism. Although they are still far from adequate, treatments for HIV infection and the opportunistic infections of AIDS have improved in recent years. For instance, all the drugs for which activists were demanding approval in 1989 are now licensed and on the market, and researchers are making progress in understanding the pathogenesis of AIDS (the mechanisms by which HIV causes AIDS). Although science appears to move at a painfully slow pace, there is some small comfort that in AIDS it is probably moving faster than in any other field.

STRATEGIES FOR TREATING HIV DISEASE

There are three possible strategies for treating HIV disease:
- attacking HIV itself, to delay or prevent its damage to the immune system;
- treating or preventing the opportunistic infections that take advantage of HIV's damage to the immune system;
- strengthening or restoring the immune system.

The best treatment is likely to involve a combination of all three approaches.

Anti-HIV interventions

Drugs have been developed which specifically target HIV at different points in its lifecycle. The first approved antiretroviral drugs have been inhibitors of HIV's reverse transcriptase enzyme (RT). Only retroviruses possess this enzyme, which is essential if the virus is to reproduce itself. Inhibiting RT prevents the production of new virus particles, slowing down its proliferation in the body. However, existing RT inhibitors are only partially effective, and can thus only delay and not prevent disease progression.

The RT inhibitors which have been the most thoroughly researched are called the nucleoside analogues. Drugs in this family include AZT (zidovudine), ddI (didanosine), ddC (zalcitabine), d4T (stavudine) and 3TC (lamivudine). Non-nucleoside RT inhibitors (also known as α-APA compounds) have also been developed, such as nevirapine and TIBOL.

Other antiretrovirals in development target different stages of the virus' lifecycle. These include:

- the binding of the virus on to human cells. HIV's gp120 envelope protein locks onto the CD4 molecule on certain cells. Possible therapeutic approaches include blocking the gp120 site either through the introduction of excess genetically engineered CD4 molecules into the body, or by stimulating antibodies against gp120 by using immunogens or therapeutic vaccines.

- the functions of specific viral enzymes and genes. For example, HIV uses an enzyme called protease in the latter stages of its replication, to break down large protein building blocks into smaller viral proteins. A number of protease inhibitors are being investigated.

Antiretrovirals as symptomatic treatment

AZT was licensed for use after it had been shown to improve the quality and probably also the length of life of people with symptomatic HIV disease. However, because HIV replication is only partially inhibited by existing antiretroviral drugs, the virus develops mutations which make it resistant to the drugs after a period of treatment. The development of resistance has been seen with both nucleoside and non-nucleoside RT inhibitors and protease inhibitors. Other anti-HIV drugs have been licensed to provide further treatment options for people who can no longer tolerate or benefit from AZT.

Antiretrovirals as early intervention

It has been established that AZT has as least short-term benefits at all stages of HIV disease. People who take it while they are still asymptomatic may experience slower disease progression in the short term. However, because of concerns about the possibility of the development of resistance and the uncertain duration of benefit, doctors and researchers are divided on when is the best time to begin antiretroviral treatment. In the USA it is common for treatment to begin once the CD4 count falls below 500; in Europe, doctors often prefer to wait until a lower CD4 count or other laboratory indicators occur, or until the development of early symptoms.

Treating or preventing opportunistic infections

Treatments for the individual opportunistic infections and tumours in HIV disease have improved dramatically since the beginning of the epidemic. It is now common for a person with

AIDS to survive a bout of *Pneumocystis carinii* pneumonia that in earlier years might well have been fatal. However, even after successful treatment of an infection, a person with AIDS remains vulnerable to that infection because of their immunosuppression and because in many cases treatment drugs only suppress, rather than eliminate, the pathogens that cause the illness. Long-term maintenance therapy, or secondary prophylaxis, is therefore often required to prevent repeat episodes of particular infections.

Prophylaxis as a form of early intervention

Primary prophylaxis aims to prevent opportunistic infections in people who are vulnerable to them because of immunosuppression. It is well established that certain conditions are only likely to occur when a certain degree of immune suppression has occurred, as measured by the CD4 count. This knowledge allows prophylactic interventions to be targeted, so that people who feel entirely healthy do not need to start taking drugs until they are genuinely at risk, and so that the risk of a pathogen developing resistance to the prophylactic drug is kept to a minimum (Table 3.1).

Table 3.1 Primary prophylaxis: the CD4 count and the timing of intervention. (Certain opportunistic infections only occur if the CD4 count has fallen below a certain level.)

CD4 range	Opportunistic infections
Any value	Tuberculosis; herpes; candida (thrush)
Below 200	*Pneumocystis carinii* pneumonia (PCP); fungal infections (e.g. cryptococcal meningitis); toxoplasmosis; cryptosporidium*
Below 100	Cytomegalovirus (CMV)
Below 50	*Mycobacterium avium intracellulare* (MAI—sometimes called MAC)

Note: *Cryptosporidiosis tends to be more severe at lower CD4 counts; at high CD4 counts it can be self-limiting (i.e. it eventually gets better without treatment).

Strengthening or restoring the immune system

Immunostimulants

Immunostimulants aim to activate the immune system either in general against all infections and tumours, or specifically against HIV. To date there is no evidence of the usefulness of such drugs in HIV disease. There is also a potential danger that by stimulating the immune system these drugs may also stimulate HIV-infected immune cells to greater replication. In principle, therefore, immunostimulants would need to be used in combination with antiviral agents to suppress viral replication while they rebuild the immune system. Another problem with many immunomodulators is that they are versions of the chemicals naturally occurring in our bodies which often cause symptoms such as fever, shivering, general malaise and other undesirable symptoms of disease, so these all occur as severe side effects of treatment with immunomodulators. Many agents have been suggested as possible immunomodulators and a few, such as α interferon, also have antiviral activity.

Immunogens ('therapeutic vaccines')

In contrast with general immunostimulants, immunogens aim selectively to activate the immune system against HIV alone. Although individuals infected with HIV will already have viral proteins in their bodies as a result of infection, the hope is that, by presenting these proteins to the immune system in a different way, the specific immune response may be augmented. For example, people bitten by rabid animals have been protected from developing rabies by subsequent inoculation with rabies virus particles. This approach gives theoretical grounds for optimism.

COMBINED INTERVENTIONS

In practice, it is likely that a combination of the various strategies described in this chapter will be employed in providing optimum treatment for HIV disease. Treatments and prophylaxes for opportunistic infections are already routinely used simultaneously with antiretroviral drugs. Many clinicians, community groups and researchers believe that the most effective way to use antiretroviral drugs will be in combination. Treatment with two or more different drugs may increase the level of antiviral effectiveness, and thus also reduce the risk of the virus developing resistance to treatment. It may also allow the use of lower doses of each drug, so lessening the likelihood of side effects.

Combinations of nucleoside analogue drugs such as AZT plus ddC or ddI are unlikely to be the most effective possible combinations, as the drugs all work in the same way. Combining a nucleoside with a non-nucleoside RT inhibitor, or an RT inhibitor with, say, a protease inhibitor or a tat inhibitor may provide the best possible antiretroviral treatment using currently available drugs. Other approaches to combination therapy might involve the concurrent use of different forms of therapeutic intervention, such as antiretroviral drugs with immunostimulators or therapeutic vaccines.

PROSPECTS FOR A PREVENTIVE VACCINE

To understand current approaches to developing vaccines against HIV, it is necessary to understand some of the characteristics of the immune system's response to HIV. HIV is unlike most other pathogens in that:

- it infects or affects key cells in the immune system, which otherwise would be involved in the fight against the virus;
- it is able to evade the normal immune response.

The humoral immune response

The humoral immune response is that part of the immune system which relies on antibodies (see pp. 15–16). It has been known for some time that antibody responses to foreign antigens can either neutralise or enhance the infection. Enhancing antibodies can actually increase the ability of HIV to infect cells. These antibodies lock on to the virus, forming complexes of virus and antibody. Laboratory studies have shown that this may make it easier for the virus to infect cells which can lock on to a different receptor, called Fc, on the antibody part of that complex. Neutralising antibodies lock on to parts of the gp120 protein on the surface of HIV, interfering with the virus' ability to bind on to CD4 and infect its target cells. Laboratory studies have shown that such antibodies are able to prevent the virus from infecting a cell for up to 30 minutes after it has attached itself to that cell's CD4 molecule. Results in chimpanzees also show that such antibodies can protect the animals from infection if they are injected with HIV. An effective vaccine against HIV would therefore aim to stimulate neutralising antibodies, but to avoid producing enhancing antibodies.

The cellular immune response

The cellular immune response is that part of the immune response which relies on CD8 cells (cytotoxic T cells). The presence of cytotoxic T cells which are able to recognise HIV antigens on the surface of infected cells and destroy those cells has been observed in people with HIV. In the case of most viruses other than HIV, these CD8 cells are the most effective means of eliminating infected cells. However, CD8 cell responses can directly contribute to the damage caused by a disease. In HIV disease, CD8 cells are believed to be the cause of inflammation in the lungs, central nervous system and lymph nodes, and also to contribute to the destruction of uninfected cells which have the HIV protein gp120 attached to their surfaces.

Memory responses

For hundreds of years it has been recognised that people who have recovered from an illness tend not to be vulnerable to the same illness again—in other words, they have acquired immunity. This is because, whenever T cells or B cells are activated by an antigen, some of the cells become memory cells. When an individual next encounters that antigen, the immune system is already primed to destroy it quickly. Vaccines work by priming the immune system before the individual is exposed to the antigen in question, so that the immune system can mount a rapid and massive response if the individual is subsequently exposed to that antigen.

Can vaccination work?

The strength of the immune response

One of the key problems faced by vaccine researchers is the relative weakness of the body's immune response to HIV. Infected people are unable to fight off the infection, and the immune system is overcome by the virus. The worst-case scenario is that vaccines will be unable to stimulate the immune system sufficiently to slow down the course of disease in infected people, or to prevent infection in those who are as yet uninfected. However, animal tests suggest that successful vaccination is indeed a possibility.

It is currently unknown whether a successful HIV vaccine would need to stimulate humoral immunity, cellular immunity or both. Greater understanding of the immune response to HIV infection should help answer this question.

The method of exposure

Vaccines that are given by injection will mainly protect the bloodstream from being infected. With any HIV vaccine it will also be important to test the effectiveness of the protective response against mucosal infection (directly into cells in mucous membranes in the anus or vagina, rather than indirectly via the bloodstream), since this is how the virus is actually transmitted during sex.

Safety

A key problem for vaccine researchers is ensuring that their vaccines are safe. In the past, monkeys have been used to test vaccines, but monkeys respond very differently to HIV and experiments really need to be done on human volunteers. Researchers can monitor volunteers' immune responses to vaccines using blood tests; however, they also need to ensure that the individual has not been infected with HIV following vaccination, which would also induce an immune response which could confuse the interpretation of test results.

Types of vaccines

Recombinant vaccines Recombinant vaccines are products of genetic engineering. They use a live, harmless vector organism into which certain genes from infectious viruses have been introduced. In the body, these viral genes produce viral proteins, but these are harmless because no other parts of the virus are present. The idea is that the presence of the viral proteins will prompt an immune response that would also recognise the real virus.

Killed vaccines Killed vaccines consist of the whole virus which has been treated with chemicals, heat or other processes to kill it and render it uninfectious. Again, the theory is that injecting it into the body will prime the immune system to recognise the real, unkilled virus. This is the principle of the Salk HIV-immunogen vaccine currently being tested.

Subunit vaccines This is a similar vaccination strategy to that of recombinant vaccines. In this case, the genes that produce selected viral proteins are grafted into bacteria, cell lines or even insects, which subsequently produce quantities of the viral protein. The protein itself is then injected into the body, to stimulate an immune response.

Synthetic vaccines Rather than using whole viral proteins, it may also be possible to use fragments of the proteins. These are called synthetic peptides—short sequences of amino acids which can be produced by chemical synthesis. However, they are only able to induce a feeble immune response.

Progress to date

Trials conducted so far have shown that all candidate vaccines tested to date evoke humoral immune responses (Haynes, 1993). Nearly all trial participants have developed binding antibodies, which 'tag' foreign antigens for recognition by other parts of the immune system. Antibodies which neutralise HIV in vitro have also been observed, but only occasionally, and usually these antibodies have been effective only against the specific HIV strain from which the vaccine preparation was derived. Virtually all vaccine trials have reported increased T cell proliferation, indicating that immunological memory has been achieved. However, the production of cytotoxic CD8 cells has only been seen in a very limited number of trial participants. Generating CD8 cells is thought to be of much greater importance than general T cell proliferation for establishing a protective immune response.

COMPLEMENTARY THERAPIES IN HIV DISEASE

Complementary or alternative therapies are used by a large number of people with HIV infection. This is probably because the therapies used in conventional medicine have failed to provide a complete cure, tend to have side effects and are perceived as only being interested in one set of cells, rather than the whole person. Holistic simply means taking into account the whole person, not just the lungs, say, but also the person's personality, social situation and work. Good doctors should do this anyway. Involvement with choosing and using a complementary therapy fosters a feeling of self-help. Possible reasons for using a complementary therapy may include having a real treatment effect on the progression of HIV or individual opportunistic infections; improving the quality of life even if the underlying HIV disease is unaffected; and establishing a more positive and assertive outlook and involvement in self-help groups. Such an approach has been shown to prolong survival in women with breast cancer, for instance.

The possible dangers of complementary therapies include

exposing oneself to potentially dangerous and untested therapies; the possibility that some therapies may interact harmfully with conventional medicines or interfere with the diet; and the fact that some therapists may charge exorbitant amounts. It is wise to be particularly cautious about practitioners who make startling claims for their therapies, or who charge substantial sums of money for them. People who are contemplating using complementary therapies are advised to talk to a self-help group about therapies which other people with HIV have found helpful, or which the group itself provides. These groups may also be able to recommend individual practitioners who are experienced in working with people with HIV and who can be trusted.

KEEPING ABREAST OF AIDS SCIENCE AND MEDICINE

Many people with HIV have shown that it is possible for someone with no medical training to become expert in understanding HIV/AIDS medicine and drug development. This learning can help individuals gain the confidence to talk to doctors and carers and get the best out of them, and to understand treatment options and know what they are entitled to. As a result, it is possible to become involved in intelligent, well-informed and constructive treatment activism, which can also lead to beneficial results for the community: more ethical trials and more urgent and functional research pursuing new directions.

HIV/AIDS community groups have had an impact upon the arrangements for trials, treatment and other health care as never before. For example, the emergence of the Community Research movement and other groups such as ACT UP has contributed immensely to better treatment and more urgent research in the USA. Constructive debate between medical professionals and community representatives needs to be encouraged and sustained (Arno and Feiden, 1992).

The tradition of passivity in health care may be strong, but there are now fresh emphases on self-help and self-education among the communities of people affected by HIV. The influence of self-help groups and the response of the medical profession has resulted in new opportunities for learning and influence. Self-help groups provide supportive information services which are sensitive to the needs of individuals with HIV, and doctors are more used to dealing creatively with complex and searching questions about treatments.

Sources of advice and information

A number of resources have been developed to help in the process of learning about AIDS science and medicine. These include accessible introductions to the important principles (such as this book); information sessions at specialist centres, such as self-help groups or clinics for people with HIV; treatment newsletters which summarise the latest medical developments in accessible language; and directories of treatments and clinical trials. Through ways such as these, people with HIV and their advocates have gained in self-confidence and knowledge. Eventually it can become reasonably straightforward to learn from the medical journals and conferences used by doctors themselves.

DEBATES ABOUT TREATMENTS AND TRIALS

The response to HIV and AIDS has been characterised by an unprecedented level of community involvement in the debates about trials and treatments. By contrast with most other areas of medicine, there has been especially lively discussion and debate about a whole range of fundamental questions, such as the priorities given to different kinds of research; the pace of research; access to treatment and care; geographical variations in service provision; the design and accessibility of trials; community consultation; and conflicts between orthodox and alternative medicine.

Research priorities

Some activists have argued that premature conclusions were reached about the nature of HIV disease following the discovery of HIV in 1983. This may have led to an oversimplified picture of the research tasks to be accomplished in order to develop therapy. In the earliest years of the epidemic, when all that was clear was that AIDS involved dysregulation of the immune system, research focused on immunology. The discovery of HIV led to the allocation of considerable research funds to virology. However, antiviral research is just one part—albeit perhaps the most challenging and problematic part—of the necessary research response to AIDS. Before 1990 the development of treatments and prophylaxes for opportunistic infections was largely neglected, and important advances such as the testing of aerosolised pentamidine for PCP prophylaxis came about only through the initiative of community-based research efforts.

More recently, it has become clear that there are many gaps in our basic understanding of the precise mechanisms by which HIV causes illness. Although it is not necessarily essential that this is completely understood for effective treatments to be developed, researchers have now placed a new emphasis on basic science as a foundation for more rationally designed therapies.

How urgently is research undertaken?

Some activists have argued that existing systems of drug development and licensing do not function at the speed necessary during a life-threatening epidemic. As a result of the constructive criticisms of groups such as ACT UP and New York's Treatment and Data Committee, promising experimental drugs are now made available to people with HIV at a much earlier stage in their development than in the past, through schemes such as Treatment IND, Parallel Track and Compassionate Use programmes. In the UK a number of so far unapproved drugs can be released to physicians on a named-patient basis.

Access to treatment and care

The relationship between the medical profession and the population at large has traditionally been an unequal one. Doctors have occupied positions of power in relation to their patients, who have often been expected to trust absolutely in medical authority.

This power imbalance has been shifting in recent years, particularly during the AIDS epidemic, as well-informed, articulate individuals have educated themselves and demanded a role in decision-making about their own medical care.

Marginalised groups within society have had particular difficulty in accessing sympathetic medical care. Surveys show that a disproportionately high number of gay men, especially in big cities, have not even registered with a general practitioner (GP), preferring to use sexually transmitted disease clinics to meet their health care needs. Many people with HIV also prefer to use specialist clinics rather than GPs. Injecting drug users have often received unsympathetic treatment from unapproving medical professionals, and women have found great difficulty in gaining respect for their wishes and opinions.

Geographical variations in experience

Historically, the majority of people with HIV in Europe have received their medical care from a relatively small number of centres of excellence. These centres have thus gained in experience and expertise in treating HIV disease, and this greater experience has been shown to translate into improved quality and length of life for their patients. Consequently, people with HIV tend to migrate both within and between countries in order to secure the best treatment. This results in a self-perpetuating situation in which skill becomes concentrated in the centres of excellence. It has been suggested that the formulation and dissemination of a minimum standard of care for HIV disease could assist in promoting the best possible care for people with HIV across geographical boundaries.

Trial design

People with HIV and their advocates have argued that clinical trials should be seen as a means of early access to promising new treatments, rather than simply as an exercise in impartial scientific research. It is argued that all aspects of a clinical trial should offer a viable treatment possibility for participants. This has led to challenges to the use of placebo drugs in certain circumstances.

The experience with the Medical Research Council's Alpha trial of ddI provided a useful case study. To avoid the need for an expanded access programme to ddI alongside the controlled clinical trials, as was the case in the USA, the trial was designed with two arms, in one of which participants were randomly assigned to receive a placebo, lower-dose ddI or higher-dose ddI, while in the other participants received either lower-dose or higher-dose ddI. Participants could choose which arm they wished to enter, and thus choose to avoid any risk that they might receive the inactive placebo rather than real ddI. All but a tiny handful chose the arm without the placebo. This should not have been surprising, as all the participants had previously taken antiretroviral treatment and now had no options other than ddI. However, the lack of a placebo arm meant that the trial was unable to establish whether ddI treatment was more effective than no treatment at all.

Representation/accessibility

There have been concerns that HIV/AIDS clinical trials have not enrolled a representative sample of women with HIV or black people with HIV to provide data on the safety and efficacy of new treatments in these populations. Most trials exclude women who are pregnant, due to ethical concerns for the welfare of the unborn child; however, some have routinely excluded all women for this reason, or have insisted that they be sterilised. Current or previous drug users have also experienced difficulty in access to trials. While scientific opinion holds that population-specific differences in the safety and efficacy of drugs are at most very uncommon, lack of access to trials also translates into lack of access to promising experimental therapies. Recently researchers have paid greater attention to securing adequate representation within trials.

Community consultation

Community consultation should be an integral part of the ongoing development of drugs. Doctors and pharmaceutical companies in the UK and elsewhere in Europe are increasingly keen to develop such links following the lessons of the United States, where people with HIV and their advocates have come to play an increasingly significant role in the development and implementation of clinical trials, because of the pressure from community groups.

In the United States input is provided into trial design, ethics and recruitment through many mechanisms, including advisory boards, organisational relationships and individual contact with researchers. Such input often produces trials which are more attractive, and thus quicker to fill with participants who are likely to remain for the duration of the study. The principal challenges are how to structure input mechanisms to make sure that they fairly represent the patient population and how to separate the sometimes conflicting needs of providing medical care versus conducting research.

Conflict between orthodox and alternative medicine

The legitimacy or otherwise of complementary and alternative medicine is an issue of vital public concern. It is increasingly recognised that clinical medicine does not necessarily provide answers to all our questions, or treatments for all our needs. Although alternative practitioners may be marginal to the mainstream medical establishment, the issues raised by alternative medicine are central if we are truly concerned with the quality of care and with people's own estimations of their health and wellbeing.

Most surveys refute the suggestion that people using alternative medicine are themselves 'alternative' or cranks: most users tend to have conditions that conventional medicine cannot cure. There is also the sense that alternative medicine may be better at coping with the social and personal dimensions of illness. It seems to allow for longer consultations and more sense of engagement with the whole person, although it is important to recognise that this may be to do with financial constraints on the National Health Service (NHS). It is important to recognise that there are some 'quacks' in alternative medicine, but we should not forget that there are dishonest and incompetent doctors too.

People with HIV should not accept being treated like children. After all, they are most likely to have the keenest sense of their own best interests. Users of complementary and alternative medicine make choices which may seem irrational to others, but these are choices that must be respected. Alternative medicine is marginal only insofar as it is used by a minority of people and often lacks official acceptance.

4

Epidemiology, transmission and testing

Simon Watney   Peter Aggleton

Epidemiology is the study of the distribution and determinants of disease within and between different population groups. It aims to identify the frequency with which particular diseases occur, as well as the characteristics of those who are infected (Barker and Rose, 1992). Epidemiology thus reveals changing patterns of disease, and may also furnish evidence concerning the modes of transmission of given diseases, as well as other information such as life expectancy and rates of disease progression. Findings from epidemiological research may be used to identify changing health care needs within the community. They can also inform the development of health education and other areas of social policy relating to health, including the direction of medical research, the planning of hospital services, the provision of community care and so on.

Major sources of data used by epidemiologists are mortality and morbidity statistics. The former are obtained from death certificates, whereas the latter are obtained from hospital records, general practitioners (GPs) and the official notification of certain infectious diseases. Occasionally, epidemiologists carry out special surveys to identify the prevalence of disease within particular populations, and to monitor the incidence of new cases. Epidemiology is thus always concerned with the health of groups of people rather than individuals, which is the province of clinical medicine. The conclusions reached by epidemiologists are closely dependent on the quality and accuracy of the data collected, and on the chosen methods of analysis. Since morbidity and mortality statistics may be incomplete or inaccurate, care should always be taken in the interpretation of epidemiological findings (Smith and Phillips, 1992).

Epidemiologists are often among the first people to be alerted to the sudden rise in the incidence (or the number of new cases within a specified period of time) and prevalence (or the current total number of cases at a specific point in time) of disease which is characteristic of the outbreak and early stages of an epidemic. They then seek to ascertain the extent of the epidemic, its causes, whom it is most likely to affect and its probable rate of future development. As a central branch of public health, epidemiology can also provide data on the basis of which appropriate funding and resources may be secured for the purposes of prevention, treatment and the identification of research needs. Epidemiology is an indispensable element within the overall process of identifying, managing and preventing epidemics. Indeed, modern epidemiology arose from the study of explosive outbreaks of infectious diseases such as cholera, typhus and typhoid (Delaporte, 1986).

Many epidemics are caused by environmental or ecological changes that favour the rapidly increased transmission of endemic diseases. The term endemic refers to the established presence of a disease, or agent of disease, within a given population. An epidemic begins with a rise in the incidence of a given disease above and beyond its usual endemic level. Sometimes, however, epidemics are caused by new diseases, as in the case of Lassa fever, first recognised in 1969, and Legionnaire's disease, first identified and named in 1976. Epidemiology plays a crucial role during an epidemic, by providing data on constantly changing patterns of disease and directing attention to changing needs, whether these are more specialised health education or more hospital beds in an affected region.

Epidemiologists are particularly interested in the risk factors associated with particular diseases, since these can form the basis for preventive measures. In the case of a new or newly recognised condition there can be special difficulties in identifying risk factors, since it may be necessary to work backwards from the medical signs and symptoms that can presently be observed, in order to identify earlier stages in the natural history of the disease. In such retrospective studies, large numbers of shared behavioural traits and patterns may be observed, and the difficulty lies in determining which of these are most significant as indicators of possible risk. However, by comparing members of a given social group who have the disease with others from the same group without it, it is possible to isolate the significant risk factors that might form the target for preventive measures. This technique is known as a *case-control study*. Epidemiologists also make use of *cohort studies*, in which they intensively study a fixed group of individuals over a period of time in order to monitor changes in their health, such as an uninfected person becoming infected with HIV or an asymptomatic person developing HIV-related symptoms, and to search for factors which correlate with these changes. In this way, the average length of time between infection and the emergence of symptoms may be established, together with an indication of those at most risk. These are often referred to as 'risk groups' or 'high-risk groups'. Epidemiological concepts of risk are, however, distinct from the notions of risk that individuals and communities may hold (Douglas, 1986).

RISK GROUPS

Epidemiologists refer to 'risk groups' to direct attention to those in most need. In this sense, a risk group is a group which is at risk and therefore in need. A high-risk group is a group at greatest risk and with the greatest needs—for targeted prevention work and other services. In relation to HIV, it has sometimes been argued that we should not talk about risk groups but rather risk behaviour, in order to clarify the nature of risks and to avoid possible stigmatisation of members of risk groups. Unfortunately, however, such an approach tends to obscure the reality of the epidemic, where it is most concentrated and devastatingly experienced.

Risk factors may change in the course of an epidemic, both for individuals and for groups. For example, the adoption of safer drug-related practices has significantly altered the extent to which, in many countries, injecting drug use is still a risk factor for HIV infection. In a similar way, the number of one's sexual partners will undoubtedly be a risk factor for HIV and other sexually transmitted diseases if safer sex is not being practised. In the early days of the epidemic, when little was known about the cause of AIDS, the number of sexual partners did play a significant role in predicting in case-control studies those who were most likely to develop AIDS. However, subsequent knowledge about HIV's modes of transmission has dramatically changed this situation, and it is important to realise that this potential risk will remain insignificant so long as the sexual behaviour of members of risk groups does not allow HIV to be transmitted. Hence health education should emphasise the distinction between the ways that HIV may be transmitted in individuals' everyday lives, and theoretical risks that may apply, or may have applied in the past, to abstract general populations. The confusion between these two levels of analysis has led to much controversy concerning who is at risk of HIV (Adler, 1987; Scott, 1993).

THE EPIDEMIOLOGY OF HIV AND AIDS

The first reported cases of AIDS occurred in the United States in 1981, following the diagnosis of *Pneumocystis carinii* pneumonia (PCP) and Kaposi's sarcoma (KS) in young gay men. Subsequent retrospective studies have shown that there were unidentified cases of AIDS in Europe, America and Africa in the late 1970s. The cause of the syndrome and its modes of transmission were not immediately apparent, and it was not until 1983 that a virus was identified and its existence made public the following year.

Subsequently the development of antibody and antigen tests has enabled sophisticated epidemiological studies to be undertaken in many parts of the world. Care should be taken in interpreting the results of such studies, since political considerations, social taboos and other factors have contributed to the underreporting of HIV and AIDS in many countries. Thus reported cases may not represent the actual incidence or prevalence of the disease. It is always important to distinguish between the epidemiology of HIV and the epidemiology of AIDS. The former concerns the changing prevalence and incidence of HIV infection, providing evidence of changing trends; the latter is concerned with patterns of disease progression, changing combinations and sequences of opportunistic conditions, and changing life expectancy rates.

The global picture

Research conducted for the Harvard-based Global AIDS Policy Coalition suggests that the magnitude of the epidemic has increased over 100-fold since AIDS was identified in 1981. By 1992 at least 12.9 million people worldwide were infected with HIV (7.1 million men, 4.7 million women, 1.1 million children) (Mann et al, 1992). The World Health Organization calculates that by the year 2000 there will be a cumulative total of 30–40 million cases of HIV infection in the world, of which more than 90% will be in developing countries (WHO, 1992). By April 1992 there had been 484 148 cases of AIDS reported worldwide to the World Health Organization. Three-quarters of these have been in North and South America, the majority in the United States, where between 60 000 and 70 000 people are currently diagnosed with AIDS each year (Karon et al, 1992). Globally, 75–90% of AIDS cases presently occur among people aged 20–40, and it is evident that many are infected in their teens. In Africa and the Caribbean men and women are affected in equal numbers. The results of numerous epidemiological studies lead to the sad conclusion that 'we should regard progression to clinical AIDS after infection with HIV as the norm rather than the exception' (Moss, 1988).

The United Kingdom

In England, Wales and Northern Ireland cases of HIV and AIDS are reported in confidence to the Communicable Disease Surveillance Centre (CDSC). Scottish figures are reported separately to the Communicable Diseases (Scotland) Unit (CD(S)U). Monitoring of the epidemic in the UK has two main components: routine surveillance and special studies. Monthly and quarterly summaries of HIV and AIDS statistics are available from the Public Health Laboratory Service. By the end of March 1993 there had been 6827 cases of AIDS among British males, of whom 4317 had died; and 514 cases of AIDS among British females, of whom 255 had died. There had also been 17 003 reported cases of HIV infection among British males, and 2468 cases among females. Of all British AIDS cases 67% have been among gay men, 12% among bisexual men and 20% among heterosexuals, including those infected through injecting drug use, blood factor treatment or blood transfusion. Gay and bisexual men also make up 66% of the cumulative total of cases of HIV among those over 15. Three-quarters of all UK cases of HIV and AIDS are in the London area. By the end of June 1992, Scotland, with a population of some 5 million people (approximately 9% of the total UK population), had recorded 313 cases of AIDS (5% of the UK total) and 1813 cases of HIV infection (10% of the UK total). Moreover, Scottish statistics provide a graphic example of regional variation and changes within the wider UK epidemic as a whole (Table 4.1)

Table 4.1 HIV-infected persons reported in Scotland by year of testing and by transmission group, 1984–1991*

Year of testing	Homosexual/ bisexual males†	Injecting drug users	Heterosexual sex only	All other transmission groups	Total (all groups)
1984	5 (2%)	153 (71%)	3 (1%)	54 (25%)	215 (100%)
1985	70 (26%)	155 (58%)	1 (0.5%)	42 (16%)	268 (100%)
1986	63 (18%)	229 (66%)	13 (4%)	41 (12%)	346 (100%)
1987	47 (16%)	156 (54%)	24 (8%)	61 (21%)	288 (100%)
1988	33 (23%)	50 (35%)	23 (16%)	37 (26%)	143 (100%)
1989	39 (31%)	45 (36%)	25 (20%)	16 (13%)	125 (100%)
1990	38 (30%)	32 (25%)	41 (32%)	17 (13%)	128 (100%)
1991	42 (28%)	42 (28%)	40 (27%)	24 (16%)	148 (100%)
Year not known	38 (46%)	16 (19%)	6 (7%)	23 (28%)	83 (100%)
Total	375 (22%)	878 (50%)	176 (10%)	491 (28%)	1744 (100%)

Notes: * As reported to the CD(S)U by 31 December 1991 and checked for duplication of reports. Positive tests for HIV-1 antibody became available for routine use in 1985; tests on sera which originated earlier than 1985 were done retrospectively during 1985.
† Includes some persons with injecting drug use and homosexual risk of infection.

(Emslie et al, 1992). Thus, the steady decline in new cases of HIV among injecting drug users since 1986 provides graphic epidemiological evidence of the efficacy of widely available needle-exchange facilities in the UK since the late 1980s, while the parallel rise in new cases of HIV among gay and bisexual men strongly suggests the need for more targeted HIV education, which has frequently been neglected (King, 1993).

HIV and AIDS figures for the UK as a whole are likely to underestimate the full extent of HIV and AIDS. Doctors may not identify AIDS as a cause of death in some cases (Boyton and Scambler, 1988). Nor is it clear what proportion of gay men are aware of their HIV status, whether negative or positive. It is apparent that by European standards the UK has a disproportionately small epidemic, although no fewer than one in five gay men taking the HIV test in London find out they are HIV antibody-positive (Table 4.2) (PHLS, 1993).

In spite of claims by some newspaper pundits that the HIV epidemic is 'a myth' or 'a hoax', epidemiological projections concerning the UK epidemic have been remarkably accurate. As the *New Scientist* notes:

> In 1992 there were 1 573 AIDS cases in the UK. The last prediction by government scientists, led by Nicholas Day at the University of Cambridge and finalised in 1989, predicted 1 600 cases for 1992, with upper and lower ranges of 950 and 2 800. The number of AIDS cases reported each quarter since 1989 has been within about 100 cases of the Day estimate each time. The newspapers are basing their claims on predictions made in 1988 and before. Those predictions, such as the Cox report were clearly wrong, based as they were on the scant data then available. No scientist has used them for almost five years.
> (*New Scientist*, 1993).

HOW HIV IS TRANSMITTED

In the early years of the epidemic there was much speculation concerning the supposed causes and modes of transmission of AIDS. It is therefore useful to distinguish between the body fluids and tissues from which HIV may be *isolated*, and the body fluids and tissues through which it may be *transmitted*. Because a micro-

Table 4.2 AIDS cases and deaths by exposure category and date of report: UK to 31 March 1993

	April 1991–March 1992		April 1992–March 1993		January 1982–March 1993			
How persons probably acquired the virus	Male	Female	Male	Female	Male	Deaths	Female	Deaths
Sexual intercourse								
between men	934	—	1118	—	5527	3506	—	—
between men and women								
'high risk' partner*	7	13	7	15	24	10	53	32
other partner abroad†	86	59	98	76	356	187	213	78
other partner UK	9	11	13	8	37	18	31	18
under investigation	1	—	7	1	9	5	1	—
Injecting drug use (IDU)	49	31	56	25	243	148	101	61
IDU or sexual intercourse between men	22	—	27	—	120	78	—	—
Blood								
blood factor (e.g. for haemophilia)	64	—	50	2	353	272	6	4
blood/tissue transfer (e.g. transfusion)								
abroad	1	4	3	6	13	8	31	19
UK	2	4	2	1	19	15	19	14
Mother to infant	9	12	14	11	38	17	45	23
Other/ undetermined	23	5	28	5	88	53	14	6
Total	1207	139	1423	150	6827	4317	514	255

Notes: *Men and women who had sex with injecting drug users, or with those infected through blood factor treatment or blood transfusion, and women who had sex with bisexual men.
†Includes persons without other identified risks from, or having lived in, countries where the major route of HIV-1 transmission is through sexual intercourse between men and women.

organism can be isolated from a particular tissue or fluid does not mean that it can be transmitted by that route. For transmission to take place, a critical quantity of the micro-organism (known as an inoculum) must pass from one person to another via a route specific to the micro-organism in question. Much of what we reliably know about the transmission of HIV derives from three different kinds of research: epidemiological studies of risk groups; sexual contact studies; and studies of households, hospitals and places of work. Such transmission studies demonstrate unequivocally that HIV may be transmitted via semen, vaginal and cervical secretions, blood and blood products, and via organ transplants. For HIV transmission to take place, three conditions must apply:

- live virus has to be introduced inside the body;
- a sufficient amount of virus needs to be present;
- HIV has to get inside the body of an uninfected person by a route which is effective for transmission to occur.

There are only four proven substantial routes for HIV transmission:

- unprotected sexual intercourse, whether anal or vaginal;
- sharing unsterilised injecting drug use equipment;
- injection or transfusion of infected blood or blood products;
- from an infected mother to her baby during pregnancy (sometimes known as vertical transmission).

Sexual transmission

HIV may be sexually transmitted from man to man (Kingsley et al, 1987; Moss et al, 1988); from man to woman (Calabrese and Gopalakrishna, 1986); and from woman to man (Fischl et al, 1987). HIV has also been transmitted via artificial insemination by donor (Stewart et al, 1985), although HIV tests are now carried out on potential sperm donors. Among gay men, anal intercourse without using a condom is by far the most significant risk, particularly to the receptive partner (Kingsley et al, 1987). There is considerable evidence which demonstrates that oral sex is safer than either vaginal or anal sex (King, 1993). This may be in part because saliva is known to contain substances which inhibit HIV (Fox et al, 1988, Fultz, 1986). There may, however, be some risk of HIV transmission if vaginal or seminal secretions come into contact with sores or cuts in the mouth. In some cases transmission takes place with the first sexual contact, while in others infection may not result even after numerous and protracted contacts (Padian, 1987).

Blood and blood products

HIV transmission via blood transfusion was first recognised in 1983 (Amman et al, 1983), and since September 1985 all donated blood in the UK has been screened for antibodies to HIV, and any infected blood has been rejected. Blood products such as the clotting factors Factor VIII and Factor IX used by people with haemophilia have also in the past been contaminated by HIV, and as a result many people with haemophilia became infected. Such blood products are now routinely treated to render them safe. HIV can also be transmitted via the sharing of syringes or needles employed by injecting drug users (see Chapter 6). Evidence for transmission via organ transplants has come from cases involving kidney transplants and skin grafts (Clark, 1987). All potential organ or skin graft donors are now routinely tested for HIV antibodies.

Mother to child

HIV may be transmitted from mother to child before or during birth, either by being transmitted across the placenta to the growing fetus or during birth from the mother's blood. There is contradictory evidence about transmission via breastfeeding: although some research has suggested that there is a possibility for transmission via breast milk, the research findings are not conclusive (Dunn et al, 1992). This ambiguity results largely because it is difficult to distinguish between infection before birth and infection during or after birth, since, even if the child is uninfected, it may carry maternal antibodies for some time after being born. This makes it difficult to determine the child's initial HIV antibody status (Semprini et al, 1987), although an increasing number of clinics now offer antigen tests for reliable early diagnosis of HIV infection in newborn children. Recent studies suggest an HIV transmission rate from infected mothers to their babies of around 20%. In a European Collaborative Study (ECS, 1992), which followed up 327 children born to HIV-infected mothers 18 months after birth, a vertical transmission rate of 12.9% was found. It is important that any risks associated with breastfeeding should be weighed up against the larger benefits this may have for mother and child, especially in the developing world. For women who are concerned about being HIV antibody-positive, it would be appropriate to discuss breastfeeding with a counsellor prior to making any decision on whether to go ahead or not.

HOW HIV IS NOT TRANSMITTED

HIV cannot be transmitted through unbroken skin; by breathing; via the mouth, so long as the skin is not broken or cut; through intact barriers such as latex condoms or polyurethane female condoms; via transplants of the cornea; by insect bites; by sharing household utensils; by social contact with people with HIV or AIDS; by animal bites; from swimming pool water, showers or washing machines; by mouth-to-mouth resuscitation; from telephones; or from lavatories. Unfortunately, groundless fears about HIV transmission have frequently been stirred up by journalists and others, who exploit irrational anxieties and phobias. We should feel confident that we understand a very great deal about HIV transmission, and that casual transmission cannot take place. Unfortunately, this confidence is repeatedly undermined by misleading mass media attention to the remotest theoretical possibilities of HIV transmission, rather than to demonstrably preventable risks.

Transmission in medical situations

Studies have calculated that the risk of HIV transmission from a needlestick injury is around 0.4% (Becker et al, 1989). This is because such small quantities of blood are generally involved in such accidents. There have been no reported cases of HIV transmission as the result of surgery; and follow-up studies of doctors and surgeons with HIV have not established any examples of HIV transmission to patients as the result of treatment. A recent study of the case of an American dentist thought to have been responsible for infecting five of his patients suggests that a failure to disinfect dental equipment was probably responsible (Cieselski et al, 1992), although another research team was unable to demonstrate any conclusive link between the dentist and his five HIV-positive patients (Debry and Abele, 1993). Concerns about adequate autoclaving or sterilising of equipment used in dental procedures in the UK have recently surfaced as a result of media reporting, but there has been no evidence of transmission of HIV via this route (Scott et al, 1993a).

HIV TESTING

It is a common misconception that a single test can indicate whether or not someone has AIDS. AIDS consists of a syndrome of some 30 potentially life-threatening conditions, which may occur in many different combinations and sequences in the wake of HIV infection. The so-called 'AIDS test' is not a test for AIDS but for HIV or, to be more precise, for antibodies to HIV. Nor does the test reveal whether or not an infected individual might develop AIDS, nor what symptoms he or she might experience. In other words, it has no immediate prognostic or predictive value in relation to clinical AIDS.

The HIV antibody test

Antibodies are produced by the body in response to infections. Such antibodies usually neutralise viruses. In the case of HIV infection, however, the antibodies produced are generally unable to neutralise the virus, which is likely progressively to undermine the immune system from within. An infected person can also infect others. Tests to detect the presence or absence of HIV can be arranged by a GP or at a sexually transmitted diseases (STD) clinic; this involves testing a small sample of blood, usually taken from a vein in the arm. Results are generally available within 2 weeks, although a growing number of clinics now provide same-day testing and results. If a test shows the presence of HIV antibodies, the person is said to have seroconverted and to be HIV antibody-positive (or HIV+). If no antibodies are found, the person is said to be HIV antibody-negative (or HIV−).

A positive test result reveals that an individual has produced antibodies to HIV infection. A negative result reveals that at the time of testing the person has not developed antibodies to HIV. Although 'false positive' and 'false negative' results sometimes occur, testing in the UK is now reported to be over 99% accurate in determining the presence or absence of HIV antibodies. A negative test result does not necessarily mean that an individual has not been infected, since there can be a delay of a matter of weeks to several months in seroconversion, or the production of antibodies. This delay, which has been described as the 'window of uncertainty', raises important questions about the appropriateness of a single HIV antibody test as a measure of an individual's HIV status.

The HIV antigen test

The HIV antigen test detects parts of the virus itself, rather than the antibodies produced in response to it. Most of the commercially available antigen tests detect the presence or absence of the core protein p24. It is also possible (although expensive and time-consuming) to test for the whole virus using HIV culture tests. The results of the antigen test may also be useful in identifying early infection, before seroconversion and the resulting production of antibodies, and in predicting the likely course of disease progression. Although an antigen test may be a sensitive way of detecting HIV infection in its early stages, when antibodies may not be detectable, there may be periods following the production of antibodies when viral components cannot be detected.

Testing is also important to epidemiologists, who can trace rising or falling patterns of new infections, reflecting effective HIV education and prevention work, or its absence. In 1989 the Department of Health announced the introduction of widespread anonymised screening of pregnant women and other social groups, in order to ascertain the prevalence and incidence of HIV in the UK. The results of such tests are not communicated to named individuals and, since names are not used, there is no risk to confidentiality (PHLS, 1993).

HIV antibody testing is a service with four primary aims:

- diagnosis: to allow individuals to find out whether or not they have been infected;
- risk reduction: to provide professional counselling about possible risks of HIV infection, whether or not the individual goes on to take the test, and irrespective of the result;
- referral: to put people with HIV in touch with medical and other welfare services, and to provide access to potentially helpful treatment drugs, or to the clinical trials of new drugs;
- stress reduction: to provide an opportunity for reassurance to the anxious, and to determine whether or not their worries are realistic.

Counselling thus plays a crucial role in relation to HIV antibody testing, both before taking the test and afterwards. Specific issues are raised for members of different social groups in relation to HIV antibody testing. For example, the position of a young gay man who took up safer sex in the mid-1980s but had unsafe sex before then is very different from that of a married heterosexual who has been unfaithful to his or her spouse, or who is afraid that his or her partner may have been unfaithful and contracted HIV. Counselling provides the best opportunity for an individual to decide whether or not to take the HIV antibody test, with fully informed consent, based on the most reliable and up-to-date medical and social information about the consequences of testing HIV antibody-positive or HIV antibody-negative.

Pre-test counselling

Pre-test counselling involves establishing whether or not an individual has been at theoretical risk of HIV infection. In the regrettable absence of demonstrably effective 'early intervention' anti-HIV drugs, testing is not usually an easy decision to take, especially for those at greatest risk. There may be benefits, such as access to specialised medical advice, prophylactic drugs which can prevent or delay the onset of such AIDS conditions as *Pneumocystis carinii* pneumonia (PCP), or the sense of taking an active decision to protect one's health. However, there may also be harm, such as the prejudice and discrimination facing those who are publicly identified as HIV antibody-positive. For heterosexual women, decisions about pregnancy may be important and these should be made in the context of the most up-to-date information about the dangers of vertical transmission from mother to baby (Scott et al, 1993a).

Post-test counselling

Post-test counselling will clearly differ for those testing HIV antibody-positive from those testing HIV antibody-negative. A negative test result should be fully explained, and not regarded as evidence of personal immunity. Members of risk groups may feel confused and even guilty, especially if close friends have previously tested positive. Such 'survivor guilt' can in some circumstances lead to the adoption of unsafe sex or unsafe drug use (Martin, 1988). A negative test result may also motivate some people to reconsider their practice of potentially risky behaviours—for example, injecting drug users may reconsider their patterns of drug use—although testing should never be regarded as a means to this end, independently of questions concerning HIV. Post-test counselling for those testing HIV antibody-positive involves extremely difficult and painful issues. It is especially important that people with HIV do not feel guilty or to blame for being infected. Nobody sets out to contract HIV. There is no evidence that testing HIV antibody-positive has any necessary consequences in relation to HIV risk reduction, although counselling is usually of value (Higgins et al, 1991). HIV antibody testing should not be thought of as if it were an alternative to, or a substitute for, education for HIV prevention.

Confidentiality

Given the controversy and widespread misunderstanding concerning most aspects of the AIDS epidemic, the guarantee of confidentiality is crucial in relation to HIV antibody testing, for without it people will understandably be unwilling to be tested and this might deny them access to vital medical information, services and other resources. Confidentiality is ensured by rules governing the use of records kept by GPs and STD clinics. Nonetheless, unscrupulous journalists and others have sometimes broken the confidentiality of people infected by HIV, and this has caused much avoidable suffering.

In April 1993 the Department of Health issued new guidelines to health care providers in the UK, including doctors. These were a response to calls in the mass media for the routine HIV testing of all National Health Service staff, in spite of the fact that there is no evidence of patients contracting HIV as a result of treatment or care within the NHS. This guidance stipulates that health care workers are expected to seek expert medical advice if they believe that they may have been at risk of HIV infection, or if they test antibody-positive, and must cease from any involvement in invasive surgical procedures. They must inform their employers via a designated person, with the understanding that this information will remain entirely confidential. If they have not performed invasive procedures, they must remain under medical supervision but do not need to inform their employer. Some companies require new employees to be tested for HIV, but this is very rare. Being tested without consent is probably illegal, and conflicts with the fundamental ethical principle of there being informed consent before all serious medical procedures or interventions, including blood tests of any kind, with the exception of anonymised screening, which has, however, been subject to some controversy.

TRAVEL AND IMMIGRATION

Since the widespread introduction of HIV antibody testing in 1985, many countries have introduced immigration restrictions designed to restrict the entry of people with HIV or AIDS. Such restrictions range from limits on tourism and short-stay visits to the denial of permanent residency. Up-to-date information on this constantly changing situation is available from the National AIDS Hotline, or can be found in the *National AIDS Manual*. It should also be recognised that discrepancies can occur between government policies and the behaviour of immigration officials, who may insult or otherwise intimidate people with HIV or AIDS in the course of their legitimate travel.

In considering the appropriateness of border controls as a means of restricting the international movement of people with HIV, the Council of Europe issued a formal statement in 1987, insisting that control measures at national borders are scientifically and ethically unjustifiable (Council of Europe, 1987). The World Health Organization (WHO) has also published an extensive report on HIV infection and international travel. It points out that since no region in the world is free from HIV infection, and given our clear understanding of HIV's modes of transmission, 'It makes little sense in public health terms, to undertake screening of international travellers using clinical aspects of AIDS as criteria for exclusion' (WHO, 1987a).

Moreover, because of the 'window of uncertainty' between infection and the production of antibodies, HIV antibody tests will not identify a newly infected person even though she or he may be capable of transmitting the virus. WHO concludes that 'HIV screening programmes for international travellers would, at best, and at great cost retard only briefly the dissemination of HIV both globally and with respect to any particular country' (WHO, 1987a).

5

Sexual health

Peter Aggleton   Paul Tyrer

In the early days of the epidemic, education about HIV and AIDS frequently took place as a one-off activity, conducted in relative isolation from other issues and concerns. Usually, people were provided with the facts about HIV, the ways in which it could and could not be transmitted, and the steps that could be taken to guard against infection. Links between HIV and AIDS and other health issues were rarely made, and workers in fields such as family planning and maternal and child health were not always willing, or sufficiently well prepared, to make the connection between HIV and AIDS and issues arising in their own areas of work. With the passage of time, this situation has changed; there is now much talk about the place of HIV and AIDS in education for healthy lifestyles, and in education for sexual and reproductive health. How and why did this situation come about, and what are its implications for the form that HIV and AIDS education should take?

THE CONCEPT OF SEXUAL HEALTH

The origins of such a move can be traced to two sources: efforts to define more clearly what is meant by reproductive and sexual health, and attempts to 'mainstream' or normalise HIV and AIDS work. There has long been debate about what is meant by terms such as 'sexual' and 'reproductive health', and even today there exists no one universally accepted definition. Some people define these terms negatively as implying the absence of sexually transmitted disease, and of unwanted pregnancy. Others adopt a more positive stance, seeing sexual and reproductive health as something enjoyable, enriching and fulfilling. The Family Planning Association, for example, sees sexual health in terms of 'being knowledgeable about reproductive health, being able to make informed choices about parenthood and sexuality, and being comfortable with one's own sexuality' (FPA, 1990). The Terrence Higgins Trust does not have one set definition but recognises that sexual health includes 'physical and emotional wellbeing, as well as the avoidance of sexually transmitted diseases, and unwanted pregnancies, with an overall focus on the practice of safer sex' (THT, 1991). The World Health Organization, which has held a number of consultative meetings on the subject, concludes that 'due to the range of individual, cultural and social differences, and the various patterns of lifestyle, social and gender roles, there can be no single definition of a sexually healthy individual' (WHO, 1987b).

For perhaps the majority of people, sexual health is about more than the absence of STDs and unwanted pregnancy, since it implies more positively the pleasures of sexual relationships and emotional closeness and the importance of taking responsibility for oneself and others. But it is in relation to these more positive aspects of sexual health that problems arise, since there exists controversy, not to say heated debate, about where, when and with whom it is legitimate for sex to take place. There are those, for example, who would seek on 'moral' grounds to restrict sexual activity to heterosexual married relationships, claiming that it is only within this context that sex should take place. There are others who hold more liberal views, arguing that there are many circumstances and relationships within which legitimate and fulfilling forms of sexual expression can occur.

Health educators have a responsibility to begin with the way things are, not with the way some people might like them to be. If they fail to do this, they run the risk of not meeting health education needs due to inappropriate messages. This means working from a definition of sexual health which recognises the diversity of human sexual behaviour and sexual desire, and which acknowledges the many different ways in which people can express themselves emotionally and sexually. Historically and cross-culturally the evidence is unequivocal: sexual health and the attainment of physical and emotional wellbeing can be achieved in a wide range of ways—through homosexual, heterosexual and bisexual relationships, and through relationships of varying characters and durations. A respect for this diversity should be the starting point for any work on HIV and AIDS, particularly if health educators want to devise messages and approaches which are relevant to all, and not just to a minority of the population.

Concurrent with the above debate there have been moves to integrate HIV and AIDS work with work in other settings and contexts. In schools and colleges, HIV and AIDS are beginning to take their place in health education and in education about personal and social relationships; in the health service there have been moves to integrate HIV and AIDS more fully within family planning and maternal and child health services; and in local authorities steps have been taken to examine the implications of HIV and AIDS for housing and social services, equal opportunities provision, personnel practices and health and safety at work. Some have seen this mainstreaming of HIV and AIDS as a bad thing, fearing a possible loss of specialist expertise and services. Others have viewed events more positively, welcoming the inclusion in HIV and AIDS work of groups hitherto marginalised.

Debates about mainstreaming have also highlighted a tension between what health professionals, including health educators, want to offer and what individuals may want to hear. HIV and AIDS are unlikely to be priority issues for communities and individuals who do not see themselves at risk. This raises important questions about the best way of meeting HIV/AIDS education needs. Is it really sensible, for example, to promote debate about HIV and AIDS-related concerns alongside topics which people do want to know about, thereby tackling two problems at the same time? The complexity of such debates cannot be entered into here. Suffice it to say that the move to integrate HIV and AIDS concerns into other fields has been progressive and sustained. It has helped establish the new context within which much HIV and AIDS education now takes place.

WORKING ON SEXUAL HEALTH

Given the multifaceted nature of sexual health, educators and trainers in this field need to be well prepared. This means beginning with an awareness of their own values, attitudes and commitments, as well as those of others. It also means recognising the existence of differing (sometimes diametrically opposed) views on sexuality and sexual health.

Education for sexual and reproductive health involves far more than the provision of facts and information. Knowing how HIV is and is not transmitted, for example, is but one step towards empowerment in the face of possible risk. Beyond information, people need to acquire the necessary skills—such as the ability to communicate openly and negotiate—by which to protect themselves and their sexual partners against HIV-related risk. For education about sexual health to be most effective it is important to attempt to develop and promote an awareness of wider issues such as oppression, gender inequality, distribution of power and cultural expectations.

The task of health educators is challenging since, if they fail to address these larger concerns, much of their work may prove ineffective. As Diane Richardson (1990) has pointed out, 'in our society it is impossible to talk about sex without talking about power'—the power to define what is right and wrong, the power to exert choice, and the power to challenge oppression and inequality wherever it exists.

Many different kinds of power may interfere with education for sexual and reproductive health. These include the power that denies women the opportunity to participate fully in sexual decision-making; the power that limits the freedom of lesbians and gay men to express their sexuality openly and without fear of attack; the power that denies those who are physically or intellectually disabled the right to a fulfilling sex life; the power that denies young people access to the information they may need to protect themselves against unwanted pregnancy and STD; and the power that encourages an understanding of black people's sexuality as being different from and inferior to that of whites. Health educators need to work to minimise the impact of these damaging forces on everyday lives by addressing the ways in which certain groups in society are scapegoated. Before this can be done, an understanding of what sexuality is, and what it entails, needs to be developed.

SEX, SEXUALITY AND SEXUAL BEHAVIOUR

First, some definitions are important. If sex denotes the biological characteristics of a person as a man or a woman, gender describes their role—the social behaviours they are expected to show within a particular society or community. Gender gives rise to behaviour which is seen as either masculine or feminine within a particular society. Sexuality, on the other hand, is more a question of identity and links closely to a person's sense of self—as heterosexual or straight; as homosexual, or lesbian or gay; as bisexual; or as neither.

It has long been known that, just as there is no necessary relationship between sex and gender (although all men are biologically male, only some are 'manly'), there are no necessary links between sex or gender or sexuality. Indeed, some of the most 'masculine' men may be gay; some of the most feminine women may be lesbian; and there are many behaviourally effeminate men with strong heterosexual identities. Regardless of the origins of these varieties and differences—and scientific opinion differs as to their causes—their existence should form the starting point for any work to promote sexual and reproductive health. How people feel about themselves sexually, or which sexual identity(ies) they have adopted, plays a large part in maintaining a sexually healthy and fulfilling life.

Lesbian and gay sexualities

Many people hold fairly stereotypical views about lesbians and gay men, who they are, what they look like, what they do. Such stereotypes usually represent lesbians and gay men as different in some way, physically, socially and emotionally. But lesbians and gay men are also viewed as inferior, their behaviour less natural and their rights less inclusive than those of heterosexuals.

The belief that homosexuality is inferior to heterosexuality gives rise to heterosexism, or the idea that lesbians and gay men are inferior to their heterosexual counterparts. Heterosexism underpins a range of divisive attitudes and beliefs, such as the idea that lesbians and gay men are child abusers; the idea that lesbians and gay men try to 'convert' others to homosexuality; and the idea that gay men cause AIDS. Young lesbians and young gay men in particular bear the brunt of heterosexism, since they may be rejected at a crucial time by their families, be subjected to bullying and other forms of violence at school and, perhaps crucially, be offered no positive role models with which to identify. The cost of such negligence is considerable, and is reflected in higher attempted and actual suicide rates among young lesbians and gay men than among their heterosexual counterparts (Remafedi, Farrow and Deigher, 1991). In the UK, and for men, the homosexual age of consent currently stands at 18, making it difficult to offer effective HIV and AIDS education to young gay men, some of whom may be particularly vulnerable to infection. This is a problem which does not exist in other countries which have lower ages of consent.

The 1980s and 1990s have seen a growing visibility of lesbians and gay men in most European societies (including those of central and eastern Europe), in North America and in Australasia. This has been witnessed in the growth of gay politics, in community newspapers and other publications, in the cinema and theatre, and in the growth of lesbian and gay bars and clubs (the gay scene, as it is sometimes called). Such events have helped establish something of a visible community among gay men and lesbians, particularly in towns and metropolitan areas. But this greater visibility has led some to claim that things have gone too far, and that more than equality is being demanded. Such views should be recognised as the expression of deep, but profoundly irrational, fears and anxieties about sexual difference. They are key aspects of the heterosexism described above.

We should recognise too that while many lesbians and gay men may feel part of a broader community, not all do so. Some live, and enjoy, relatively isolated lives, preferring that their sexuality remain a private matter. Others, like some of their heterosexual counterparts, prefer to demonstrate their sexuality more openly, at work, on the street and through their social pursuits. A person's sense of self as a lesbian or gay man can vary too: there are those for whom sex is a central part of life; there are others for whom sex may be less important. There exists no single lesbian or gay identity to which an individual may aspire. Rather, there is a variety of possible identities open to those with same sex desires, and it is this variation which should be the starting point in education for sexual health, not the assumption that all lesbians and gay men are the same.

Heterosexuality

Just as there is no single lesbian or gay identity, there is no single heterosexual identity or lifestyle. However, because heterosexuality is accepted as a 'normal' and 'natural' part of life, most people rarely consider what it means to be heterosexual. It is almost as if heterosexuality is so natural that it need never be thought or talked about. This silence makes it difficult to think about the more sinister side of some of the institutions, traditions and practices linked to heterosexuality (e.g. forced marriage, the sexual division of labour within households and the double standard of morality applied to women's and men's sexual behaviour). It also reinforces stereotypes about heterosexuality which may be very difficult for some people to live up to—stereotypes that tell us what it is natural for women and men to do in heterosexual relationships, about the emotions they should feel and the manner in which they should behave.

Such views encourage us to think about heterosexuality in an overly uniform way, as if all heterosexuals have the same desires and interests. This is clearly not the case: heterosexual men differ from one another in their desires, as do heterosexual women. As Jeffrey Weeks (1986) has pointed out, heterosexuality is a diverse phenomenon, embracing 'rape as well as loving relationships, coercion as well as choice... it covers a multitude of sexual practices from intercourse in the missionary position to oral and anal intercourse'.

For many people though, there is a taken-for-grantedness

about heterosexuality which makes it difficult to move beyond stereotypes that would have us understand relationships in terms of 'boy meets girl, they fall in love, they marry, have children, and live happily ever after....' This is clearly not the way the world is, at least for heterosexuals in the UK, many of whom will remarry at least once in their lifetime and a significant number of whom are likely to have one or more extramarital affairs. Indeed, it could be argued that the hallmark of heterosexuality is its ability to resist solid definition. In education for sexual and reproductive health, this means beginning with the real experiences of heterosexuals, be they young or older, and not with what we might wish to be the case.

Bisexuality

A not insignificant number of people have sex at least once with a man and at least once with a woman in the course of their lifetime, but does this necessarily mean that the person concerned is bisexual? In one sense it does, behaviourally at least. But in another sense it does not, since their fantasies while having sex may not have been congruent with the sex of the partner at the time, nor will that same person necessarily think of him or herself as being bisexual. This highlights once again the fluidity of sexual identities, since there is no necessary relationship between a person's sexual behaviour and how they see themselves sexually. Although bisexual behaviour has been with us for a very long time, a bisexual identity is a much more modern phenomenon, with perhaps the majority of behaviourally bisexual women and men seeing themselves as either heterosexual or lesbian or gay.

In the popular imagination, bisexuality is usually associated with men and what men do, rather than women, highlighting society's refusal to acknowledge women as sexual beings when men are absent. At various times, bisexuality has been stereotyped as something of a glamorous lifestyle, being embraced by some popular musicians, among others. Since the advent of HIV and AIDS, however, bisexual men have been singled out for blame, being widely perceived as the major 'bridging group' for infection between gay men and heterosexuals. The evidence for such an assertion is inconsistent and inconclusive. Indeed, there is some evidence to suggest that bisexual men are particularly likely to practice safer sex with male partners, thus making transmission of HIV to female partners less likely (Boulton, Schramm Evans, Fitzpatrick and Hart, 1991).

SEX AND RISK

When the contraceptive pill became freely available in Europe in the 1960s, many believed that the main risk linked to heterosexual penetrative sex—an unwanted pregnancy—was no longer a problem. For a large number of people, worrying about the safety of sex, and therefore 'negotiating it', became a thing of the past. In spite of this, sex has seldom, if ever, been risk-free.

Until the advent of antibiotics, sexually transmitted diseases (STDs) such as syphilis were much feared, and in the 1970s viral infections such as herpes were heralded as a major threat in many parts of the world. Hepatitis B is also an infection which can be transmitted sexually, with serious consequences for those who have not been vaccinated. Although many STDs can be easily treated if diagnosed sufficiently early, some may be difficult to detect, and for others treatment may require the use of powerful and expensive antibiotics.

For those who have grown up in circumstances in which the contraceptive pill is readily available and where access to STD services is both confidential and free, it has come as a shock to learn that sex is once again risky. Faced with this realisation, it is little surprise that many have fallen back on three classic strategies by which to avoid dealing directly with a problem: denial ('the problem does not exist'), displacement ('the problem has nothing to do with me') and delay ('I'll change my behaviour one day, but not right now').

Denial is most clearly seen in recent media claims in the UK and elsewhere that there is no major AIDS epidemic, despite the fact that by late 1992 in Africa, Asia and Central and Southern America more than 11 million people were already infected, the majority through heterosexual sex (WHO, 1993). Displacement can be witnessed in efforts to claim that HIV affects only particular groups—Americans in the Philippines, westerners in China, Thais in Myanmar, Indians in Bangladesh, and Africans, gay men and injecting drug users in the UK. Delay can be seen most graphically in the slowness with which many governments responded to the epidemic when it first became apparent in the early 1980s.

SAFER SEX FOR ALL

Because HIV is present in blood, semen, cervical and vaginal secretions, and because it has been shown to be transmitted during sex which involves the penetration of the vagina or anus, safe sex is any sexual activity which does not involve penetration. Safer sex, on the other hand, is the term used to describe sexual activities in which efforts are made to reduce the risk of infection, through the use of condoms, for example.

Much emphasis has been given to the construction of lists of sexual activities, ranked in terms of increasing risk, as if it is possible to predict with mathematical accuracy the risk linked to a particular sexual act. This is not the case. What it is important to emphasise, however, is that (i) sex without penetration poses no threat of infection and (ii) condoms, when properly used, significantly reduce the risk of HIV transmission during penetrative sex. Table 5.1 summarises instructions on proper condom use.

The female condom, or Femidom, is a relatively new kind of protection for use during penetrative sex. This polyurethane disposable condom is inserted into the vagina and held in place by an inner ring which rests against the cervix, and an outer ring which stays outside the body. When used correctly and inserted before penetration takes place, it offers some protection against STDs, including HIV, and may offer some women additional feelings of control. As with the male condom, opinions vary about its acceptability and the female condom is available only in a limited number of countries at present.

Although it is generally agreed that oral sex poses less of a risk than vaginal or anal sex, there is a possibility of HIV transmission if semen or vaginal secretions come into contact with abrasions or cuts in the mouth. Condoms can make oral sex even safer, and

CORRECT CONDOM USE

To use a condom properly, the following steps should be followed:

1. Carefully open package so the condom does not tear. Do not unroll the condom before putting it on.
2. If not circumcised, pull the foreskin back. Squeeze the tip of the condom and put it on the end of a hard penis.
3. Continue squeezing the tip of the condom while unrolling it until it covers all of the penis.
4. Always put a condom on before entering your partner.
5. After ejaculating (coming), hold the rim of the condom and pull the penis out before it becomes soft.
6. Slide the condom off without spilling the semen inside.
7. Dispose of the condom by throwing it away with other rubbish.

Remember:

- Do not use grease, oils, lotions or Vaseline as a lubricant with condoms. These will make condoms break. Use a water-based lubricant such as 'K-Y jelly'.
- Use a new condom every time you have sex.
- Store condoms in a cool, dry place. Do not use condoms which are old or damaged. Look for the 'Kitemark' on condom boxes to guarantee they meet appropriate safety standards.
- Do not use a condom if the package is broken, the condom is brittle or dried out, the colour is uneven or changed, or if the condom is unusually sticky.

Source: World Health Organization (1992) *Guide to Adapting Instructions on Condom Use*, Geneva, WHO.

---

flavoured condoms are now available. For oral sex on women, small squares of latex known as dental dams can offer protection against getting vaginal or cervical secretions in the mouth. Alternatively, a condom can be cut along its length and used to provide a suitable barrier.

Some people claim that too much emphasis has been given to condom promotion in safer sex education. They point to evidence that not everyone finds sex with penetration pleasurable (Kahn and Davis, 1982), as well as findings suggesting that the failure rate of condoms when used for family planning purposes may be as high as 5–10%. Much of this failure is explained by non-compliance with the steps outlined in Table 5.1. Because of this, and because some people may find condoms unacceptable on moral or other grounds, alternatives to penetrative sex should figure prominently in safer sex education. These include stimulating your own or a partner's genitals with fingers or hands; massaging, stroking and cuddling each other; rubbing your body closely against the other person; licking, passionate kissing and so on. But the human sexual repertoire is wider than this, and the advent of HIV and AIDS has encouraged discussion about many sexual activities hitherto considered exotic or esoteric. These include the use of sex toys such as dildos, which are perfectly safe so long as they are not shared and are washed carefully after use, as well as practices such as watersports (sex involving urine), scat (sex involving defecation) and rimming (mouth to anus contact). While many of these activities pose little threat of HIV transmission, there may be other health hazards involved. It is important to remember when offering advice about HIV-related risk not to confuse facts about the risk of transmission with moral judgements about the acceptability of particular kinds of sexual behaviour. The *National AIDS Manual* contains an extensive and non-judgemental discussion of the health risks associated with different sexual activities, including those described above (Scott et al, 1993b).

Safer sex and disabled people

Although the principles of safe and safer sex described above provide general guidelines for HIV-related work to promote sexual and reproductive health, they may need to be adapted when working with particular groups, or when devising health education messages for specific audiences. When working with disabled people, for example, it may be necessary to confront the prejudice and discrimination such individuals face before discussing sexual behaviour and safe(r) sex. Much of this discrimination has its origins in parents' and carers' attempts to deny the sexuality or sexual needs of disabled people. Many disabled people enjoy full and happy sexual lives; others would like to have similar opportunities, but find that the accommodation in which they find themselves has only single beds, or does not allow sex on the premises. Privacy can also be an issue when locks are not provided on bedroom doors. People with learning disabilities may be denied sexual health education entirely because the issue of consent is perceived (inappropriately) as problematic. In such situations it may be necessary to tackle more general issues before addressing HIV and AIDS-related concerns. Specialised educational resources are available to support work in this field.

Safer sex and black and minority ethnic communities

The sexual and reproductive health education needs of black and minority ethnic communities are diverse. While the need for prejudice-free information remains, HIV-related messages need to be presented in ways which are culturally and linguistically accessible. This means more than translating safer sex materials into a different language. It involves a sensitivity to the circumstances in which sex, injecting drug use and other activities are talked about within a particular community, and a readiness to engage with such concerns in HIV and AIDS-related work (Dada, 1992).

Racism must be confronted in HIV and AIDS education within black and minority ethnic communities. From early in the epidemic, black people have been scapegoated as a consequence of the suggestion that AIDS 'came' from Africa (Kitzinger and Miller, 1992). It is understandable that some black groups have concluded that HIV and AIDS awareness is a tool for promoting racism, and have distanced themselves from involvement. Other black groups have found themselves having to undertake immense amounts of work, particularly since some white HIV/AIDS educators and trainers have decided that it would be 'racist' for them to promote safer sex within the black and minority ethnic communities. Here, there can be productive opportunities for the co-facilitation of training courses and for a greater sharing of the responsibilities that the HIV epidemic brings with it.

Safer sex and heterosexual men

Education to enhance the sexual and reproductive health of heterosexual men has been most usually conspicuous by its absence. In the UK, much HIV and AIDS awareness has emphasised women's responsibility for sexual safety, implying overtly or otherwise that heterosexual men may be unable or unwilling to take the initiative when it comes to safer sex. Such an approach is not only patronising but unrealistic, in that it fails to address the control that men have over the circumstances in which sex occurs, and the form that it takes. To suggest that heterosexual women should 'insist' that their partners use a condom when having sex is to deny the physical danger women may face when attempting to do so with husbands, boyfriends and other male partners. It may be more appropriate to argue for health education activities that encourage critical reflection on the ways in which male power limits both men's and women's potential for expression, sexually and otherwise.

Sexual health of lesbians and gay men

Finally, something needs to be said about the sexual and reproductive health needs of lesbians and gay men, and the place of HIV and AIDS education in meeting such needs. Since the early days of the epidemic, lesbians and gay men have had a central role to play in education for prevention and in the provision of HIV-related care. In some circumstances their actions have been particularly visible, as in some AIDS service organisations and some health and local authorities. This involvement has led some to suggest that the HIV and AIDS-related sexual health needs of lesbians and gay men are largely met: that lesbians are a 'low-risk' group, for example, and that gay men have largely changed their behaviour in response to the epidemic. Recent evidence leads us to question both of these assumptions.

Lesbians will be at the same risk as other women if they share injecting equipment or have occasional sex with a man. Artificial insemination by donor may pose special risks if the semen has not been tested for HIV and other STDs; and the little research which has been undertaken on woman to woman transmission suggests that, whereas sex between women poses only small risks, it is dangerous and irresponsible to suggest that there is no risk at all (Lyle, 1992). Additionally, many women's health services have been developed with heterosexual women in mind, and some lesbians may feel unwilling to seek treatment and advice from services which they fear will be unwelcoming or oppressive.

Gay men have been consistently blamed for 'causing' the HIV epidemic in the developed world, and politicians, commentators and the popular press have advocated isolation, quarantine, tattooing and even extermination as solutions to the threat they supposedly cause (Watney, 1987). Gay men not only have to live with the threat of HIV in their own lives and those of their friends and lovers, but also with the homophobia that often goes unchallenged in society. It is perhaps not surprising that recent research suggests an increase in unsafe sex among some gay men, particularly those who are younger. The causes of these changes in behaviour are many, but they include a relative neglect of prevention activities for gay men by health authorities and AIDS service organisations throughout the 1980s (King, Rooney and Scott, 1992). The increase in the numbers of men engaging in unsafe sex may also be the result of some gay men using a knowledge of their HIV antibody status to negotiate contracts with partners about the circumstances in which safe(r) and unsafe sex (which may not, in the circumstances, involve a risk of HIV transmission) takes place.

What is crucial in work to promote the sexual health of lesbians and gay men is a willingness to tackle divisive fears and prejudices about homosexuality, for in the absence of this, few lesbians and gay men can develop the self-respect that heterosexual men and women take for granted. Without this self-respect, there can be little hope for healthy decision-making on sexual and reproductive health issues.

6

HIV, AIDS and drug use

Brian Pearson

There may be a variety of ways in which the use of drugs is related to HIV and AIDS. For example, it is a common assumption that when people drink alcohol they are less likely to have safer sex. This view is too simple, as the relationship between alcohol and sexual behaviour is more complex and variable and no clear causal connection has been established between the consumption of alcohol and unsafe sexual practice (Plant and Plant, 1992). What is clear is the relationship between injecting drug use and HIV and AIDS, both in terms of the numbers of people infected with HIV through injecting drug use, and the association between injecting drug users and HIV and AIDS in the popular consciousness. This chapter therefore concentrates primarily on the key concern of injectable, rather than other, drugs.

In many European countries as well as in the United States, the initial spread of HIV among gay men was followed by a second wave among injecting drug users and their sexual contacts. In some cities seroprevalence among injectors reached high levels very quickly: 60% in New York, 53% in Milan, 51% in Edinburgh. By the end of 1991, and in the countries of the European Community, infection via injecting drug use had been responsible for 35.2% of non-paediatric cases of AIDS, and in 1991 reported new cases of AIDS in injecting drug users exceeded those in gay men. In Italy and Spain drug injectors now make up over 50% of AIDS cases. The position in the UK is less extreme, with the exception of parts of eastern Scotland, but provides no ground for complacency. At the end of March 1992, injecting drug use accounted for 7% of all AIDS reports in England and Wales; for Scotland the corresponding figure was 37%. Injectors constituted 11% of HIV-positive reports in England, Wales and Northern Ireland and 62% in Scotland (PHLS, 1992).

ATTITUDES TO DRUGS AND DRUG USERS

The use of psychoactive substances to alter states of consciousness is an almost universal feature of human societies (Weil, 1986), as is the existence of strong beliefs about precisely which drugs it is acceptable to use and about the circumstances in which their use is appropriate and allowed. Easier international travel and the ingenuity of chemists have combined to present a wide and growing menu of psychoactive substances to potential consumers. In western societies alcohol and (to a decreasing extent) tobacco are tolerated, even valued, despite the immense health burdens their use imposes. But drugs such as heroin, cocaine, amphetamine, LSD, ecstasy and cannabis are generally disapproved of and their use heavily sanctioned. Public attitudes to such drugs and their users are strong, highly negative, usually tinged with fear and anger and often resistant to rational argument.

Attitudes to drugs are the result of many factors (Griffiths and Pearson, 1988) which cannot be explored in depth here. Negative attitudes and beliefs about drugs are commonly transferred to those who use them. Users become stereotyped as 'addicts' and 'junkies', labels which allow the automatic imputation of additional undesirable attributes: viciousness, irresponsibility, weakness of the will, laziness, amorality, sickness and criminality, for example. Drug users, especially injectors, form one of the most stigmatised sections of society, a fact that poses problems for the design and delivery of effective treatment and prevention responses. Habits of secrecy and distrust of authority may be deeply ingrained in injectors, sustained by the ambivalent or hostile attitudes they may encounter when they come forward for help. The Advisory Council on the Misuse of Drugs (ACMD, 1988) recognised the need to reform public and professional attitudes, since attitudes and policies that result in drug users remaining hidden will impair the effectiveness of measures to reduce the risk of HIV infection.

A BRIEF HISTORY OF DRUG USE IN BRITAIN

In the 19th century the use of opium-based preparations as a form of self-medication was common among working-class people and, from the time of De Quincy and Coleridge, members of artistic and literary circles experimented with drugs. In 1917, suspicions that prostitutes were supplying cocaine to British troops led to stricter control under Regulation 40B of the Defence of the Realm Act. Further legislation followed the First World War, but despite the Dangerous Drugs Acts of 1920 and 1923, recreational use of cocaine continued in the 1920s among sections of the upper classes (Berridge, 1988). Morphine and heroin users between the wars were predominantly middle-aged and middle-class. Over half were women, and many had become dependent as an unintended result of medical treatment, or had easy professional access to opiates. Neither they nor the 'smart set' dabblers in cocaine constituted self-conscious drug-using subcultures: it was not until the 1960s that the 'drug problem' in its modern guise was born.

The 1960s saw dramatic changes in the nature and extent of drug use. Socially disapproved drugs like cannabis, amphetamine and LSD became a recognised part of the new youth culture. A new generation of heroin users also emerged. The majority were young men: they were drawn from all socioeconomic classes, defined themselves by and through their drug use and were prone to 'turn on' their friends.

These developments gave rise to great public concern. Legal controls were tightened, a process culminating in the passing of the Misuse of Drugs Act (1971) which laid down severe penalties for possessing, manufacturing and trafficking in almost all commonly 'misused' drugs. But, if the legal net was spread wide, the medical response was narrowly focused on heroin use. Following the recommendations of an interdepartmental committee chaired by Lord Brain, specialist clinics, known as drug dependence units (DDUs), were set up. They concentrated almost exclusively on the treatment of opiate dependence, a bias characteristic of medical services to the present day.

The British response to drug use has always oscillated between the twin poles of treatment and punishment. Users are seen alternatively as the victims of some rather ill-defined illness and as wilful deviants, a contradiction nicely embodied in the Brain Committee's characterisation of the 'addict' as 'a sick person, provided he does not resort to criminal acts'. The Rolleston Committee of 1926 had established that it was, under certain circumstances, a permissible form of treatment to prescribe heroin (or in later years methadone, a long-acting and less euphoriant substitute) on a more or less open-ended basis. In practice, though not necessarily in intention, this was the approach that has become known as maintenance. But by the early 1980s the demands of rising numbers of patients upon inadequate resources, and disillusion with long-term prescribing as a means of promoting positive change, had left most clinics unwilling to prescribe except as part of a time-limited detoxification programme. Immediately prior to the recognition of HIV among drug users, the pursuit of abstinence had become the prevailing medical orthodoxy.

Opiate use increased steadily throughout the 1970s, then rose dramatically at the beginning of the 1980s. The number of opiate users has continued to rise since then: some two-thirds of those notified to the Home Office are reported to inject. The end of the decade saw concern about the rising use of 'crack' cocaine, but the most significant development was the increasing popularity of the so-called 'dance drugs' such as ecstasy, amphetamine sulphate and LSD.

The official response was again twofold: on the one hand, new legislation was passed, increasing the penalties for drug trafficking; on the other, central government funding made possible a large expansion of drug services, both statutory and voluntary.

THE DIVERSITY OF DRUG USE

The term drug use subsumes a wide range of different activities, with different importance and meanings for those involved. For most people, drug use is simply one enjoyable element in their lifestyles and they experience few if any problems as a result. Such a recreational style of use is typical of most drinkers, or cannabis smokers, for example. Any problems that do occur (occasional bad experiences with the drug, spending too much money, social disapproval, brushes with the law etc.) can be dismissed as a price worth paying for the good times the drug provides. Some users, however, become physically or psychologically dependent on their drugs: they drift into a position where drug use, for whatever reason, becomes central to their lives and identities, which become organised around the acquisition and consumption of drugs.

DRUG-RELATED PROBLEMS: MEDICAL, SOCIAL AND LEGAL

Drug users do not inevitably experience problems as a result of their use, nor should the fact of use allow the assumption to be made that there is some pre-existing pathology. Nevertheless, substances which are both pharmacologically powerful and socially disapproved can, on occasion, lead to a variety of difficulties, physical, psychological, social and legal.

Drugs can impair mental and physical functioning in many ways, including intoxication, overdose, drug-induced psychoses, paranoia, physical and psychological dependence. The route of administration is also important: injecting is easily the most hazardous. Needle sharing and other unsterile or poor injection techniques can expose users to a variety of hazards, quite apart from HIV, including hepatitis B and C, septicaemia, endocarditis, ulcers and abscesses, collapsed veins and gangrene. Drug use is sometimes destructive of family and social life, leading to family breakdown, homelessness, loss of employment and children being taken into care. The need to finance a habit may lead to involvement in burglary, shoplifting, prostitution or drug dealing. Even the most casual and problem-free user may fall foul of the provisions of the Misuse of Drugs Act; in 1990 nearly 45 000 people did so, mostly as a result of minor possession offences.

The heavier the involvement with drugs, the greater the

likelihood of experiencing drug-related problems. Problems tend to be more frequent among injectors: not only is injection inherently risky, it is also more common among users who are physically or psychologically dependent upon drugs, and whose social and economic circumstances are unstable, all factors which militate against the adoption of HIV risk reduction practices.

Injectors often encounter and react to HIV risks within a context of already existing problems. HIV prevention and treatment approaches need to allow for the barriers to receiving and acting upon risk reduction and health advice posed by the coexistence of these other problems.

SPECIALIST SERVICES FOR DRUG USERS

Services for drug users are provided by both statutory and non-statutory agencies. Every Regional Health Authority possesses at least one drug dependence unit, usually situated within a psychiatric hospital. Headed by a consultant psychiatrist, DDUs vary in their staffing, resources and treatment policies. Primarily oriented to treating opiate dependents, most will prescribe oral methadone, either as part of a detoxification programme or on a longer-term basis. Sometimes heroin or other injectables will be prescribed, but a few clinics refuse to prescribe at all. In-patient beds specifically for treating drug users are comparatively rare: most in-patient detoxification takes place in general medical or psychiatric wards.

A more informal and less medically oriented service is provided by non-statutory street agencies. As the name implies, they aim to offer easy access to advice, counselling and referral. Many have links with local doctors to provide primary health care and prescribing options.

Community drug teams (CDTs) act as a primary contact point for people with drug problems. These vary in size, but typically include nurses and social workers among their staff. CDTs may offer a prescribing option, either through a clinical placement or by arrangement with local GPs. Many CDTs and street agencies run needle and syringe exchanges and provide free condoms and advice on safer sex and drug use.

Residential rehabilitation houses offer an environment designed to help residents to achieve and sustain a drug-free way of life. Almost all insist on new residents being drug-free immediately prior to entry. The content of the rehabilitation programme varies from house to house, some adhering to the 'concept house model', which combines a hierarchical work regime with the techniques of growth psychology, others having a Christian orientation, while yet others run more relaxed and informal programmes. The continued existence of these facilities is currently under severe threat, due to changes in government arrangements for financing care in the community. There are also some 20 fee-paying private sector rehabilitation houses for those with drug or alcohol problems.

Mainliners is a service for drug users set up specifically in response to HIV. Positively Women, although having a wider brief, pioneered and remains an invaluable source of advice and support for women drug users. In London the Griffin Project, run by Turning Point, provides residential and nursing care for drug users with HIV-related illnesses.

INJECTING DRUG USE AND HIV TRANSMISSION

Drug users who share needles, syringes and other injecting paraphernalia such as spoons run the risk of contracting or transmitting HIV: sharing is an extremely effective way of spreading the virus. The risk of infection will vary with the frequency of sharing, the number of people one shares with and the prevalence of HIV infection in the particular sharing network. The risk can be eliminated by ceasing to share and reduced by sharing less often, sharing with fewer people and cleaning equipment before use.

The Advisory Council report, *AIDS and Drug Misuse, Part 1* (ACMD, 1988), concluded that 'the advent of HIV requires an expansion of the definition of problem drug use to include any form of drug misuse which involves, or may lead to, the sharing of injecting equipment. This in turn means that services must now make contact with as many of the hidden population of drug users as possible'. This implies an increased emphasis on education and public health approaches to drug users and suggests two goals: reducing sharing among those who already inject, and reducing the rate at which new recruits turn to injecting. In practice, there has been an almost exclusive concentration upon existing injectors, and attempts to reduce the incidence of new injectors are rare. Targets have been set under the *Health of the Nation* initiative which envisage reducing the percentage of injectors who report sharing injecting equipment in the previous 4 weeks by at least 50% by 1997, and by at least a further 50% by the year 2000 (from 20% in 1990 to no more than 10% in 1997 and no more than 5% by the year 2000).

No one knows how many injectors there are in the UK. Any estimate must be based on informed guesswork rather than firm figures: in 1988 the Advisory Council Report referred to above estimated the number at between 37 000 and 75 000. A reasonable guess might now put the total near the upper limit of this range.

Before injectors became aware of the risk of contracting HIV, syringe sharing was widespread. Research in England, Wales and Scotland found that 62% of respondents had shared in the previous 4 weeks, with higher figures for Scotland (76%) and for those not in contact with services (Stimson, Alldritt, Dolan, Donoghoe and Lart, 1988). Sharing took place for a variety of reasons, the most obvious and common being difficulty in obtaining equipment; others included social sharing between friends or partners and a disinclination to carry needles and syringes in case one was stopped by the police.

RISK REDUCTION AND HARM MINIMISATION

At any given time, most drug users either do not want or do not feel able to stop. The aim of harm minimisation, therefore, is to reduce as far as possible the amount of harm associated with drug use (on an individual, communal or societal level, depending on the context). Giving up drugs altogether is not ruled out, but it is not the only or main criterion of success. Minimising drug-related harm and HIV risk reduction are closely connected as compatible, but not identical, activities. An injector who has successfully adopted HIV risk reduction practices by stopping sharing and practising safer sex might still be at risk from other drug-related harms. HIV risk reduction is thus best attempted within the wider context of harm minimisation.

For harm minimisation and risk reduction strategies to be effective, they must reach as many drug users as possible. Only a minority of injecting drug users are in contact with services: a figure of one in five is often quoted, but the proportion no doubt varies with time and place. The need to attract the invisible majority has caused existing services to modify their practice and new areas of work to be opened up. Drug services have had to take on a public health role as well as their traditional commitment to the welfare of the individual. The Advisory Council report, *AIDS and Drug Misuse, Part 1* (ACMD, 1988), declared unequivocally that 'the spread of HIV is a greater danger to individual and public health than drug misuse'.

The emphasis has shifted away from abstinence towards reducing the level of drug-related harm in general, and the risk of HIV transmission in particular. This has led to active attempts to attract and retain contact with injecting drug users through 'user-friendly' services which present as few obstacles to potential users as possible, and which provide tangible goods, such as clean injecting equipment or a methadone prescription, without requiring an often insincere commitment to stopping use as an entry ticket into the service.

7

Living with HIV and AIDS

Peter Scott   Peter Aggleton   Paul Tyrer

Earlier chapters have examined the epidemiology, transmission and prevention of HIV and the medical aspects of care for people with symptomatic disease. This chapter focuses on people living with HIV disease and their health-related needs. It goes without saying that a wide range of individuals have now been directly affected by HIV, either by living with the disease itself or by having friends, lovers or relatives who are so affected. In one sense, therefore, people with HIV and AIDS come from all walks of life. This is because HIV is transmitted by penetrative sex and the exchange of blood and blood products, and from mother to baby. These are activities that at least some people from any social group engage in, irrespective of their social background or identity.

However, contrary to what we might hear, HIV and AIDS do not affect different groups of people equally. Two of the more memorable public health slogans from the epidemic are 'HIV/AIDS Affects Everyone' and 'AIDS Does Not Discriminate'. They have been used in campaigns all over the world. In one sense such messages are both helpful and accurate, but in another they are not. The first message, for example, aims to highlight two rather distinct phenomena: the social harm which extends beyond those actually infected with the virus, and the possibility that HIV disease may in time affect groups other than those presently at special risk. But, more worryingly, the phrase 'HIV/AIDS Affects Everyone' also implies that the epidemic is undifferentiated in its effects—that all communities and groups are equally affected. This is not the case, as we have seen earlier (Chapter 2) and as we will see again in this chapter.

The second message, 'AIDS Does Not Discriminate', is similarly misleading: although it directs attention to the human origins of prejudice against people living with HIV or AIDS, it also implies that HIV is some kind of 'equal opportunities' virus, affecting everyone equally. Epidemiologically this is nonsense. As with almost any other pathogen, HIV affects some groups more than others, and will continue to affect different groups in the population disproportionately into the foreseeable future.

When thinking about HIV and its effects, we should therefore guard against being too easily seduced by images and understandings that oversimplify the ways in which a collection of overlapping micro-epidemics (see Chapter 4) have different impacts on individuals and communities. Although in some sense we are all living with HIV and AIDS, the reality of this experience differs considerably, depending upon the person affected, the community or group to which she or he belongs, and the health resources at their disposal. This is not to imply, however, that the epidemic is unpatterned in its effects. Some groups are more vulnerable than others, both to infection and to subsequent HIV and AIDS-related prejudice and discrimination. In Europe, North America and Australia these include the conventional 'risk groups':

- gay and bisexual men—who constitute approximately 80% of people with AIDS in the UK, and approximately 60% of all newly detected cases of HIV transmission, and who may be under constant pressure to hide their sexual and emotional relationships;
- injecting drug users—the next largest group affected, and who may risk both physical and emotional harm in a society where many injectable drugs are illegal;
- people with haemophilia—who have to face not only two medical conditions (HIV disease and haemophilia) but also the knowledge that they were infected through contaminated blood products.

Also vulnerable are black people—who may be socially disadvantaged through a lifetime's experience of racism, and who may have had to cope with cultural dislocation and insecurity about their immigration status; and women—who may be living in social situations where they have limited control over their social and sexual options, or who may be having to look after children in unsupported circumstances.

THE EXPERIENCE OF LIVING WITH HIV OR AIDS

People discover that they have HIV or AIDS in many different circumstances. It may be through an HIV antibody test while the individual is completely well, or as a result of symptomatic illness which may or may not carry the label, or diagnosis, of AIDS. As discussed earlier (Chapter 2), the majority of people with HIV at any one time do not, in fact, know they have HIV. Some people may have half-expected to be diagnosed HIV antibody-positive, for example if a lover has already been diagnosed this way, but for others the news may be completely unexpected. Others may not know that they are infected until after they are already ill.

A wide range of emotional responses is possible, depending on an individual's previous attitudes to, or beliefs about, health: shock, feelings of guilt, frustration, fatalism, anger at the health education they did not receive, or health care precautions that were not taken, and so on.

MEDICAL CONSEQUENCES

Because HIV disease is ultimately a life-threatening condition, it should be recognised that everyone with HIV and AIDS lives with the constant stress of knowing that they may become seriously ill. The signs and symptoms that others take for granted as evidence of a cough or 'flu may for them be the first evidence of more serious, and possibly life-threatening, disease. One of the uppermost fears that can affect people with HIV disease is that of becoming weak or infirm so that there is a loss of control and independence in everyday life. Housing that is perfectly adequate at present may become impossible to manage in if, for example, there are too many stairs and no lift. There may also be fears of losing physical or mental capacities, of pain, hospitalisation and death.

Given that AIDS is a syndrome made up of many possible medical conditions (see Chapter 2), people can experience the medical course of HIV disease and AIDS in many ways. Someone with early Kaposi's sarcoma on their skin may have to come to terms with signs of their illness that are visible to themselves and others, even though their outlook for the next few years may be otherwise relatively healthy. On the other hand, someone with an acute attack of *Pneumocystis carinii* pneumonia (PCP) will have an immediately life-threatening condition requiring urgent hospital treatment.

Most people with HIV and AIDS can be either well or sick at any one time. There is no single experience of HIV or AIDS because a number of different conditions can develop at different stages of the disease. Although there are laboratory markers of infection which are useful in medical research and treatment, there is no way of predicting what is going to happen to a particular individual. Equally, there are long-term survivors — people who have been living with HIV disease for up to 10 years. Medical science has not yet established why some people with HIV stay healthier for much longer than others, but as time goes by and increasingly more is known about HIV disease, the greater are our grounds for optimism about improving treatments. Although there remains no cure for HIV disease, treatments for the various opportunistic infections have considerably improved and continue to improve. However, there is a balance to be struck between the degree of optimism we can have about the likely course of HIV disease in an infected individual and the speed of medical progress. It can be both dangerous and cruel to exaggerate about treatments that are not available at present, or which are either wholly untried or experimental.

In the first decade of the epidemic there was a tendency to draw a firm distinction between HIV and AIDS in order to offer solace to those with HIV by reassuring them that there was a very good chance that they might not develop AIDS. Although such a strategy was well meaning, it tended to write off people with AIDS as if they had crossed a line from which there was no going back. It also left an increasingly large number of people with HIV infection in a peculiar limbo, being denied access to some of the albeit limited services available to those with an AIDS diagnosis, and with little accurate information about the nature of their condition or realistic expectations for the future.

It is increasingly recognised that such an approach is at serious odds with the notion of disease progression to be found in much of the medical literature. Although orthodox medicine offers no cure, it can make available treatments that improve the quality of life by treating opportunistic conditions and delaying immune system damage. To encourage people with HIV infection to believe that they stand a good (or even reasonable) chance of never developing AIDS may, moreover, be to encourage their alienation from the very services that statistically have been shown to delay both disease progression and the onset of opportunistic conditions. Attempts to reassure at all costs may also prevent the individual from making long-term plans which may improve the quality of their life or trigger the kind of denial which, when punctured, leads to greater problems later.

SOCIAL CONSEQUENCES

The overwhelming testimony of people with HIV or AIDS is that they are subject to continuing prejudice in many different ways. To develop an adequate understanding of what it means to live with HIV disease, we must learn to appreciate the extent to which those living with HIV are living with other people's prejudices. Although there are signs of improvement in some general attitudes towards people with HIV, it is probably fair to say that what has been achieved is no more than the creation of 'safe havens' where people with HIV need not experience so directly the discrimination and harassment they encounter elsewhere. At its worst, this prejudice surfaces as blame. What could be described as medieval attitudes still prevail in many quarters, with those affected being blamed for the health circumstances in which they find themselves. In few other areas does such victim blaming still occur. So powerful and relentless is this tendency to blaming that it is all too easy for self-blame to develop, leading to lowered self-esteem and further health problems.

Even more common is a kind of passive prejudice: a casual process which writes off people with HIV disease as if they were under an immediate death sentence. Many people are surprised to learn that perhaps the majority of people with AIDS spend most of their time living in the community. The vast majority of people with HIV can have many years of good health. But one of the things which distinguishes this epidemic from all others is that very little public education has taken place to encourage tolerance, care and compassion for people with HIV. Indeed, quite the contrary, people with HIV have been either ignored or featured only as a warning to others in perhaps well-intended but misguided health promotion efforts to prevent HIV transmission. The negative effects of this have been compounded by mass media messages implying that safer sex is a matter of choosing partners carefully. Not only is this ineffective advice for preventing HIV transmission: it has a demonizing effect by implying that people with HIV are somehow bad people to be distinguished from those we might love or care for. Is it really surprising, then, that there has been little room in most public discussion for solidarity?

It would be wrong to imply that people with HIV experience this kind of prejudice and discrimination uniformly. Some may have been told that they have HIV without proper counselling and support. For others, a misplaced fear of AIDS may result in unjust treatment in housing, such as when landlords and neighbours find out that someone has AIDS and react with panic and prejudice. Similarly, although there is no risk of HIV transmission in the workplace, people with HIV or AIDS who tell their employers still may risk losing their jobs. It is also common for the confidentiality of people with HIV to be disrespected, and for improper disclosure to lead to harassment and even violence. The effects of such discrimination may not end, even with death. Lovers, friends and families of people who have died with AIDS are often 'protected' by death certificates and obituaries which disguise the cause of death. Although this may spare them extra pain at the time they are grieving, it perpetuates the vicious cycle that implies that there is something shameful or immoral about having had HIV disease.

In our concern for those affected by a disease, it is perhaps natural to focus on the individual. However, we cannot begin to understand all of a person's needs unless we are also aware of how the epidemic has affected communities or social networks. Because HIV in adults is transmitted through unprotected penetrative sex and shared injection equipment, the epidemic has affected most people with HIV in the form of a double blow: not only are they themselves infected, with all that that involves, but it is likely that some of the most important people in their lives may be infected too. A range of anxieties may be involved. A gay man with HIV, for example, may be well but caring for a lover who is ill, infirm or dying, and on top of that have to cope with the fear that the same thing will befall him. Conversely, someone who is ill may have a lover who is HIV antibody-positive, and fear for their future wellbeing. For some, there may be additional feelings of guilt at the possibility that they infected their lover.

There may be multiple bereavements to cope with too. By a cruel irony, this may sometimes be worse for long-term survivors who have attended various support or self-help groups and found that new friends have also died. For gay men in particular, there has been the fear of devastating and catastrophic harm to their community as a whole, a community based after all on a shared sense of sexual identity. The invention and widespread adoption of safer sex among gay men has helped temper this. Nevertheless, it is important to understand that, because a number of years can elapse between infection and the development of symptoms, those who have been practising safer sex for many years are still falling ill now, having been infected many years ago.

Parents are likely to have particular fears and concerns for their children. For some parents, especially those who inject drugs, there may be anxiety about losing custody of their children, and there will be inevitable concerns about who will look after the children in the event of death. There is a chance that children born to mothers with HIV may themselves have HIV, and such children will have special and differing needs. Not the least of these arise from the fear and hostility they may encounter from the parents of other children in school settings, even though the risk of transmission is remote.

For some people, especially if they are young, HIV may mean a very real fear of losing their independence. For example, some young gay men may effectively become imprisoned away from their friends and communities if, when ill, they are looked after in their parent's home because the law, and social or health care services may not understand who their real sources of support may be: namely, their elective community rather than their biological family.

For some people, important social networks will often have revolved around social recreations involving sex or drugs, such as alcohol. For the person with HIV to be isolated from these networks, especially at first, may create a sense of having lost the most important pleasures in their life. Many people also experience a feeling that the way they relate to their own body has totally and irreversibly changed. Although safer sex and safer drug use may go some way to rectifying this sense of dislocation, we should not underestimate the difficulties for many people in coming to terms with safer sex. Commonly, people with HIV will go through weeks, months or even years of feeling that spontaneous and carefree sexual and emotional fulfilment is a thing of the past.

For anyone with HIV, there are likely to be extra problems in their relationships. For lovers and married couples, there will inevitably be difficult decisions: whether the other person should be tested; what kind of sex to have within the relationship; what kind of sex to have outside the relationship. For women in particular, there will be fear of transmission to their baby if they become pregnant. Some women decide to bear children, others decide not to; but either way there will be a great sense of loss.

Anyone's experience of the effects of a disease is profoundly affected by how it affects their closest friends and family. This is not unique to HIV/AIDS; however, in at least one important respect there is a completely different state of affairs. With almost any other disease, family and friends tend to rally round, and sympathy and assistance flow without prompting and without recrimination. In the case of AIDS this may not be the case.

Disclosure of a person's HIV status may also involve disclosure of that person's sexuality or drug use or dependency to relatives or close friends. Parents and friends may be faced with information about an individual's lifestyle, sexuality or drug use that they find difficult to understand and accept. Alternatively, they may, opportunistically, treat AIDS as some kind of vindication of their side of a long-buried or still-festering family disagreement and take an 'I told you so' approach. A diagnosis of AIDS might provide a handle on which to hang long-standing resentment of a sexual partner, for example. All this means there are likely to be different problems for different individuals, depending upon the kinds of relationships they had before diagnosis.

A person with HIV or AIDS may also be faced with difficult questions about their new identity. Are they the same person as before, but with a potentially life-threatening medical condition? Or do they have to become someone new, in response to an unprecedented epidemic? A constant irritant for people with HIV is that others may want to score points at their expense, to deny their individuality and use them as some sort of 'lesson'. At its worst this will consist of brutal 'moralising' by those who take comfort in others' discomfort; but it can also be irksome to be treated with a well-meaning reverence simply for being a person with HIV.

It is understandable that, given a life-threatening condition, people will seek to find what comfort they can. This may mean reviewing all available options and reconsidering what is most important in life. Unfortunately, there is a thin line between this and the kind of evangelism that presents AIDS as some sort of opportunity to stop and reassess everything in one's life, and almost presents it as a blessing in disguise. This is deeply offensive and far from the truth so far as people's experience is concerned.

Some people will want to make HIV/AIDS a very important part of their life. This means coming to terms with its effect on their lives by fighting back, perhaps as part of a new and unprecedented development, through a culture of activism rather than as patients. Others have made a different choice. Although much advice is focused upon empowering people to take an active part in decisions about their care, treatment and life choices, we need to respect choices that people make which do not match this approach. Some people will still decide that taking as little interest in HIV as possible and entrusting decisions to their health care providers is the best course. In effect, they have made an active decision not to have the rest of their lives organised by the need to fight a virus. In practice, most people with HIV fit somewhere between these two extremes.

Throughout the world there have been attempts to construct a kind of 'rainbow alliance' of the different communities most affected by HIV and AIDS. This has been important in working towards solidarity between different groups in the population, while responding to differing needs with appropriate services. Since the mid-1980s there has been a steady movement towards separate support groups and services, and thus separate AIDS or HIV identities. Women with HIV had lacked a specifically defined community with which to identify. There was also the mistaken belief that AIDS organisations only provided services to gay men. Thus it was particularly important to set up specific support and self-help groups and assert the identity of women with HIV. Conversely, injecting drug users had a history of different kinds of social networks and a different range of separately funded agencies throughout the country. Some gay men have felt that they too have lost out to a general HIV/AIDS identity. Often they encounter a degree of anger when they demand the same services that other groups receive.

SERVICE PROVISION

In many parts of the UK today, people with HIV have access to a range of services provided by organisations such as the NHS, local authorities, self-help group, charities and other voluntary agencies, both HIV specific and non-specific. Some services, such as acute medical treatment for opportunistic infections, are only available within the clinical setting provided by health service clinics and hospitals. Although such diversity is to be welcomed, competing and overlapping services may be uncoordinated and can lead to the same service being provided by organisations with different practices and policies. Duplicated provision may extend choice, but a more coordinated, centralised approach might help deliver a broader range of services. In addition, such 'choice' needs to meet the requirements of women, black people and drug users more effectively, since until recently much of the service provision on offer has focused on the needs of gay men.

Although choice exists in some places, other parts of the country, particularly rural areas, are often unable to offer specialised services: care is provided instead within generic health and social provision settings, which are less accustomed to dealing with the problems that come with HIV infection. Naturally, the throughput of service users greatly affects the kind of service that can be provided, and therefore where someone lives will often determine whether the care provided reflects the most advanced developments. For example, in *Gay Times* (June 1992), journalist Kris Kirk wrote of how his incipient CMV retinitis was misdiagnosed in rural Wales because the clinicians had never dealt with such a case before: this error led to his becoming blind.

Access to clinical trials is also dependent on geography, since these are available almost exclusively in bigger cities, with the best variety to be found in London. Equally, for those undiagnosed but concerned, the 'same-day testing' services offered by some of the larger centres may prove more appealing than local testing services, where results may take up to 2 weeks.

People with HIV are proving to be an extremely sophisticated group of health care consumers, as recent pressure group successes with drug therapy trials has shown, and their activism has brought benefits in terms of service standards which generic health care could learn to emulate. Such sophistication means, for example, that many people will travel some distance in order to access the services they want, if they can afford to do so and if their health allows. Innovations such as the buddy/befriender system, the excellence of specialised HIV centres/hospices, the extensive use of complementary therapies and general patient self-advocacy are just some of the results of this activism and are very much to be welcomed.

The government's NHS reforms

The government's NHS reforms have led to perhaps the biggest health care reorganisation since the establishment of the NHS. In previous years, District Health Authorities were responsible for managing hospitals within their boundaries and had centralised control over how local health care services were rationed and structured, including overall responsibility for budgets. The reforms have created instead NHS Trust Hospitals, independent of district control, with their own budgets. Trusts provide services which are then 'purchased' at District level: this purchaser/provider split, as it is known, encourages Trusts to compete against one another for patients, and has established a market economy health care system.

HIV services are developing within this new context: prevention, for example, has traditionally been coordinated from within district services such as health promotion, which are increasingly being passed on to Trusts, or set up in their own right as Directorates, because of the difficulty in squaring districts' purchaser role with the provision of general services. HIV service providers may therefore find it more difficult to influence the general development of policy, planning and service delivery, since for the most part they are no longer working within centralised authorities. HIV Prevention Coordinators may be forced to become either purchasers or providers, and leave behind their earlier combination of the two, since the current system makes no allowance for such dual roles.

Further reform in the future, perhaps with mergers of districts or boundary changes, may see Trusts competing without reference to geographical barriers. Although this may make it easier for people with HIV to seek treatment where they choose, it may have an impact on general HIV service provision, with some Trusts specialising in other fields and deciding to offer no HIV services at all.

The success of the Community Care Act (1992) will to a large extent depend on whether community providers are sufficiently resourced. Either way it should at least enable more people with HIV to receive care at home, where they are surrounded by people they know and where they are buffered from institutional prejudice. It is likely too that the acute sector of the NHS will look more towards community providers in order to meet some of its patient needs, and we can perhaps expect NHS managers to take a more ambitious approach to community care in years to come.

The reforms have also created GP fundholders, family doctors who opt to manage their own budgets. This has led to fears that treatment for people with HIV may be withheld because such GPs have financial limits on prescribing. However, the government has stressed that more expensive drugs should not be withheld if there is a need and that any such requirements will be taken into account when allocating budgets. There is an additional concern, however, that the expense of treating HIV and its related illnesses may convince some GPs to refuse to allow people with the virus to register on their lists in the first place.

The NHS reforms have encouraged change in other sectors too. The voluntary sector now plays a prominent role in providing a range of services which have traditionally been the responsibility of Local Health Authorities, for example, grant giving or meals delivery. As ever more needs are expressed by vocal advocacy groups, many previously uninvolved organisations are finding themselves in a position to play a part in AIDS care.

Medical care

People with HIV currently receive much of their care from small specialised or large generic units, some of which are involved in trials of anti-HIV or anti-opportunistic infection therapies. A range of services is on offer—again, dependent on the unit's facilities and experience, but prophylactic treatments, cell counts and other ways of monitoring are widely available. In fact, because of AIDS activism, people with HIV will in some places receive the most sophisticated, forward-thinking care available in the NHS.

In addition to, or sometimes instead of allopathic (or medical) treatments, many people use one or more complementary therapies. These range from disciplines such as herbalism, acupuncture and homoeopathy through relaxion techniques, yoga, massage and aromatherapy to art therapies and mystic or spiritual therapies. Although these therapies are to an extent still in the specialist domain, some are now becoming more part of mainstream health care: as well as being provided free at a number of HIV centres, hospitals are starting to employ a wider range of professionals (aromatherapists, for example) for generic care.

Community care

Perhaps the most complex patchwork of providers can be seen in the home. District nurses from the local Community Health Care Trust can rub shoulders with home carers from the local authority; social workers, GPs, buddies/befrienders, specialist nurses and others may also have a part to play, not forgetting perhaps the most important carers—partners, friends and families. The Community Care Act has meant that health care workers can provide an ever-increasing range of services in the home—for example, proactive health organisations have trained community nurses so that they can administer some drug and prophylactic treatments at home, which can make a huge difference to quality of life. In some places, multi-agency HIV teams work together to provide the range of services that people in their area require, including very practical needs—for instance, shopping, cooking, cleaning or walking the dog. Buddies, or befrienders (people who volunteer to offer practical and/or emotional support to people with HIV and AIDS), may also be involved in some of this work.

HIV centres

When care at home is proving difficult, specialist HIV centres can offer integrated packages of care and support to people with HIV and their significant others. Having opportunities for partners and relatives to stay over is an important aspect of this, as is provision for children whose parent(s) may not be able to care as effectively as in the past. Services have greatly expanded in order to meet the broad range of needs of those infected. What were more or less hospices when they were established in the 1980s have now developed into residential and day care units, often resembling community centres with activities such as drama workshops, painting and creative writing on offer. Facilities such as legal advice, help with benefits and general information are also available, alongside services giving psychological and spiritual help.

Some people self-refer to an HIV centre to give themselves and their carers a break after a period of illness. Others use a centre as a hospice when they are coming to the end of their lives, perhaps returning home in their last few days to be able to die there. Some others use drop-in or day care facilities to meet particular needs. The flexible, holistic approach of these centres is an excellent model of care to be emulated.

Welfare, financial and housing services

There are a number of reasons why people with HIV may need extra financial help. Particular household items can make a huge difference to quality of life, but are often out of reach to someone on state benefits: a washing machine, for example, is an essential requirement for people with night sweats or chronic diarrhoea. Some individuals may have to leave work because of illness, or because of prejudiced or ill-informed employers, leading to a huge drop in income and lifestyle possibilities. Those in this position will need advice on how to make the most of the benefits system, which can provide a perplexing number of welfare payments, and other avenues of financial help. Citizens' Advice Bureaux (CAB) will be able to offer some help, and individual CABs may offer HIV-specific advice sessions. Local and national AIDS helplines can provide guidance too, and may in some areas be best placed to give appropriate advice. In addition, ever more HIV voluntary agencies are setting up their own trust funds to give one-off payments for essential items or for adaptations to accommodation. The Social Fund, part of the benefits systems, can also give one-off grants, but these are very limited and loans, which may prove difficult to repay, are now more the norm. There is a better chance of receiving a grant if the person discloses their HIV status, but some may understandably be reluctant to do so.

Equally, if a person needs rehousing, proof of HIV status may be required in order to get the help necessary. However, this may not be enough, since it is up to the discretion of individual local authorities as to whether even a diagnosis of AIDS constitutes a priority need for housing. If rehousing is agreed, the person concerned may have a long wait before permanent accommodation is made available, and because of this some people have died before being properly housed. The range of problems that someone with HIV-related illnesses may face should be reflected in the type of housing provided, but this is not always the case and wholly unsuitable temporary accommodation may be offered instead. Asking for advice from local voluntary sector groups about how to approach issues of rehousing may be a good first step, since they may be able to refer to specialist HIV housing agencies, either through local authorities or housing associations.

Emotional support and counselling

Naturally, the most important source of emotional support is from care given by lovers, families and friends. Increasingly, however, the phenomenon of multiple loss, where someone has lost many friends to AIDS, can mean that others play a central role in providing that care. This applies equally where someone has no links with family, either because of location or because of family breakdown. Buddy or befriender services are again important here, also providing respite for any primary carer by taking on some of the emotional needs. Buddy training must therefore be rigorous and in-depth; some may even befriend more than one person at a time, and therefore such services need to build in proper support mechanisms for carers in order to function effectively.

Specialised counselling is also available from the public sector: psychologists are on hand in some clinics, offering clinical counselling for all HIV-related mental problems; HIV counsellors, health advisers and social workers may also be involved in meeting some support needs.

Education

There is an ever-increasing range of information material produced by people with HIV, HIV service organisations and medical bodies focusing on myriad issues, including treatments, medical ethics, patient rights and housing and welfare issues. This takes the form of newsletters, leaflets or books, often nationally or internationally distributed and many free of charge to people with HIV. Some of these publications are very influential, organising extremely effective lobbying. HIV centres provide opportunities for people with HIV to learn more about the plethora of issues they may have to deal with, and some Health Authorities are also taking a more active role in this area. Charities too are doing excellent work in information provision, in particular the *National AIDS Manual*, which gives regular updated access to the widest range of issues. Perhaps the most useful educational contribution has been from people with HIV themselves, sharing information about drug treatments and trials, ways of coping and ways of making the most out of life: much of this takes place within support groups or at conferences or other meetings. Equally, some have talked openly about their experiences on television, radio and in daily newspapers and on educational videos, helping to demystify and destigmatise HIV and AIDS for everyone else. The impact this has had on public perceptions of the epidemic and of those with HIV should not be underestimated.

CONCLUSIONS

Throughout this chapter, as elsewhere in this book, the aim has been to demystify aspects of the HIV epidemic, particularly its impact on the lives of individuals and communities most affected. This is essential if genuine education about HIV and AIDS is to take place, and care services are to be more thoughtfully planned.

This work has attempted to clarify areas which are central to an understanding of HIV and AIDS from both scientific and social perspectives. It has concentrated on key issues and has attempted to convey the main findings of recent research relevant to health educators. There is now extensive literature on HIV and AIDS; the references listed at the end of this book provide guidance on further reading on the many challenging issues for health educators concerned with HIV and AIDS.

References

ACMD (1988) AIDS and Drug Misuse, Part 1, *Report by the Advisory Council on the Misuse of Drugs*, HMSO, London.

Adler, M. (1987) The development of the epidemic, in M. Adler (ed.) *The ABC of AIDS*, London, British Medical Journal, pp. 1–3

Aggleton, P., Moody, D. and Young, A. (1992) *Evaluating HIV/AIDS Health Promotion*, London, Health Education Authority.

Aggleton, P., Young, A., Moody, D., Kapila, M. and Pye, M. (eds) (1992) *Does It Work? Perspectives on the Evaluation of HIV/AIDS Health Promotion*, London, Health Education Authority.

Amman, A. et al. (1983) Acquired immunodeficiency in an infant: possible transmission by means of blood products, *Lancet*, i, pp. 956–958.

Arno, P. and Feiden, K. (1992) *Against the Odds: the Story of AIDS Drug Development, Politics and Profits*, New York, Harper Collins.

Bagnall, G. and Plant, M.A. (1991) HIV/AIDS risks, alcohol and illicit drug use among young adults in areas of high and low rates of HIV infection, *AIDS Care*, 3, 4, pp. 355–361.

Barker, D.J.P. and Rose, G. (1992) *Epidemiology for the Uninitiated*, London, British Medical Association.

Becker, C.E., Cone, J.E. and Gerberding, J (1989) Occupational infection with HIV, *Annals of Internal Medicine*, 110, 8, pp. 653–656.

Berridge, V. (1988) The origins of the English drug "scene" 1890–1930, *Medical History*, 32, pp. 51–64.

Boulton, M., Schramm Evans, Z., Fitzpatrick, R. and Hart, G. (1991) Bisexual men: women, safer sex and HIV transmission, in P. Aggleton, P. Davies and G. Hart (eds) *AIDS: Responses, Interventions and Care*, London, Falmer Press.

Boyton, R. and Scambler, G. (1988) Survey of general practitioners attitudes to AIDS in the North West Thames and East Anglian regions, *British Medical Journal*, 296, 20 February, pp. 538–540

Burt, J. and Stimson, G.V. (1990) *Strategies for Protection: Drug Injecting and the Prevention of HIV Infection, Report to the Health Education Authority*, London, Goldsmiths' College.

Calabrese, L.H. and Gopalakrishna, K.U. (1986) Transmission of HTLV-III infection from man to woman to man, *New England Journal of Medicine*, 314, p. 987.

CCETSW (1992) *Improving Social Work Education and Training, 11, HIV and AIDS in the Diploma in Social Work*, London, Central Council for Education and Training in Social Work (CCETSW).

CDC (1992) 1993 Revised Classified System for HIV Infection and Expanded Surveillance Case Definition for AIDS among Adolescents and Adults, *Morbidity and Mortality Weekly Reports*, 41, RR-17.

Cieselski, C., Marianos, D., Chin-Yih, Ou, Dumbaugh, R., Witte, J. et al. (1992) Transmission of human immunodeficiency virus in a dental practice, *Annals of Internal Medicine*, 116, 10, pp. 798–805.

Clark, J.A. (1987) HIV transmission and skin grafts, *Lancet*, i, p. 983.

Connor, S. and Kingman, S. (1989) *The Search for the Virus: the Scientific Discovery of AIDS and the Quest for a Cure*, Harmondsworth, Penguin Books.

Council of Europe (1987) Recommendation No. R(87), 25 November.

Dada, M. (1992) *Multilingual AIDS: HIV Information for the Black and Minority Ethnic Communities*, London, Health Education Authority.

Debry, R.W. and Abele, L.G. (1993) Dental HIV Transmission? Letter. *Nature*, 361, 6414, p. 691.

Delaporte, F. (1986) *Disease and Civilization: the Cholera in Paris, 1832*, Cambridge, Mass., Massachusetts Institute of Technology Press.

Donoghoe, M.C. (1991) Syringe exchange: has it worked?, *Druglink*, January–February, London, ISDD, pp. 8–11.

Douglas, M. (1986) *Risk Acceptability According to the Social Sciences*, London, Routledge and Kegan Paul.

Dunn, D.T., Newell, M.L., Ades, A.E. and Peckham, C.S. (1992) Risk of HIV transmission through breast feeding, *Lancet*, 340, pp. 585–588.

ECS (1992) Children born to women with HIV-1 infection: natural history and risk of transmission, *Lancet*, 239, pp. 1007–1212.

Emslie, J. (1992) Monitoring the spread and impact of HIV infection in Scotland, 1982–1991, *AIDS Scotland*, Issue 7, Glasgow, Communicable Diseases (Scotland) Unit.

Evans, B., Sandberg, S. and Watson, S. (eds) (1992) *Working Where the Risks Are*, London, Health Education Authority.

Family Planning Association (1990) *Manifesto for Sexual Health and Family Planning*, London, Family Planning Association.

Fischl, M.A., Dickinson, G.M., Scott, G.B., Klimos, N., Fletcher, M.A. and Parks, W. (1987) Evaluation of heterosexual partners, children and household contacts of adults with AIDS, *Journal of the American Medical Association*, 257, 5.

Fox, P.C., Wolff, A., Yeh, C.K., Atkinson, J.C. and Baum, B.J. (1988) Saliva inhibits HIV infectivity, *Journal of the American Medical Association*, 116, pp. 635–637.

Fultz, P.N. (1986) Components of saliva inactivate HIV, *Lancet*, 2, 1215.

Gallo, R. (1991) *Virus Hunting*, New York, Basic Books.

Griffiths, R. and Pearson, B. (1988) *Working with Drug Users*, Wildwood, Aldershot.

Haynes, B.F. (1993) Scientific and social issues of human immunodeficiency virus vaccine development, *Science*, 260, 5112, 1273–1279.

Higgins, D.L. et al. (1991) Evidence for the effects of HIV antibody counselling and testing on risk behaviours, *Journal of the American Medical Association*, 266, 17.

Kahn, S. and Davis, J. (1982) *The Kahn Report on Sexual Preferences*, New York, Avon Books.

Karon, J. M., Buchler, J.W., Byers, R.H., Farizo, K.M., Green, T.A., Hanson, D.L. and Rosenblum, L.S. (1992) Projections of the number of persons diagnosed with AIDS and the number of immunosuppressed HIV-infected persons—United States, 1992–1994, *Morbidity and Mortality Weekly Reports*, 41, RR-18.

King, E. (1993) *Safety in Numbers: Safer Sex and Gay Men*, London, Cassell.

King, E., Rooney, M. and Scott, P. (1992) *HIV Prevention for Gay Men: a Survey of Initiatives in the UK*, London, North West Thames Regional Health Authority.

Kingsley, L.A., Kaslow, R., Rinaldo, C.R., Detre, K., Odaka, N., Van Raden, M., Detels, R., Polk, V.F. et al. (1987) Risk factors for seroconversion to human immunodeficiency virus amongst male homosexuals, *Lancet*, i, 345–349.

Kitzinger, J. and Miller, D. (1992) "African AIDS": the media and audience beliefs, in P. Aggleton, P. Davies and G. Hart (eds) *AIDS: Rights, Risk and Reason*, London, Falmer Press, pp. 28–52.

Kramer L. (1990) *Reports from the Holocaust*, London, Penguin Books.

Levy, J. (1993) Pathogenesis of human immunodeficiency virus infection, *Microbiological Review*, 57, 183–289.

Lyle, R. P. (1992) No evidence for female-to-female transmission among 960 000 female blood donors, *Journal of Acquired Immune Deficiency Syndromes*, 5, 853–855.

Mann, J., Taratola, D. and Netter, T. (eds) (1992) *AIDS in the World*, Cambridge, Mass., Harvard University Press.

Martin, J.L. (1988) Psychological consequences of AIDS related bereavement among gay men, *Journal of Consulting and Clinical Psychology*, 56, 856–862.

Moss, A.R., Bachetti, P., Osmond, D., Krampf, W., Chaisson, R.E., Stites, D., Wilber, J., Allain, J.P and Carlson, J. (1988) Seropositivity for HIV and the development of AIDS or AIDS related condition: three-year follow-up of the San Francisco General Hospital Cohort, *British Medical Journal*, 295, 745–750.

New Scientist (1993) The Numbers Game, 1 May, Comment, p. 3.

Padian, N. (1987) Male to female transmission of human immunodeficiency virus, *Journal of the American Medical Association*, 258, 6, 788–790.

Pantaleo, G., Graziori, G. and Fauci, A.S. (1993) The immunopathogenesis of human immunodeficiency virus infection, *New England Journal of Medicine*, 328, 5, 327–335.

PHLS (1992) PHLS AIDS Centre—Communicable Disease Surveillance Centre and Communicable Diseases (Scotland) Unit. Unpublished quarterly surveillance tables No. 15, March 1992.

PHLS (1993) PHLS AIDS Centre—Communicable Disease Surveillance Centre and Communicable Diseases (Scotland) Unit. Unlinked anonymous monitoring of HIV prevalence in England and Wales: 1990–1992, *Communicable Disease Report*, 3, 1, R1–R11.

Plant, M. and Plant, M. (1992) *Risk-Takers: Alcohol, Drugs, Sex and Youth*, London, Tavistock/Routledge.

Remafedi, G., Farrow, J. and Deigher, R. (1991) Risk factors for attempted suicide in gay and bisexual youth, *Paediatrics*, 87, 869–975.

Richardson, D. (1990) *Safer Sex: the Guide for Women Today*, London, Pandora Press.

Scott, P. (1993) Beginning HIV prevention work with gay and bisexual men, in B. Evans et al. (eds) *Healthy Alliances in HIV Prevention*, London, Health Education Authority, pp. 148–165.

Scott, P. and Alcorn, K. (eds) (1993a) *National AIDS Manual, Volume 1: Topics, Section B* (Summer edition), London, NAM Publications Ltd.

Scott, P. and Alcorn, K. (eds) (1993b) *National AIDS Manual, Volume 1: Topics, Section C* (Summer edition), London, NAM Publications Ltd.

Semprini, A., Vncetich, A., Pardi, G. and Cossu, M.M. (1987) HIV infection and AIDS in newborn babies of mothers positive for HIV antibody, *British Medical Journal*, 294, 610.

Smith, G.D. and Phillips, A.N. (1992) Confounding in epidemiological studies: why "independent" effects may not be all they seem, *British Medical Journal*, 305, 757–759.

Stewart, G.J., Cunningham, A.L., Driscoll, G.L., Tyler, J.P., Barr, J.A. and Gold, J. (1985) Transmission of human T cell lymphotropic virus type III (HTLV-III) by artificial insemination by donor, *Lancet*, ii, 581–584.

Stimson, G.V., Alldritt, L., Dolan, K.A., Donoghoe, M.C. and Lart, R. (1988) *Injecting Equipment Exchange Schemes — Final Report*, Monitoring Research Group, Goldsmiths' College, University of London.

Terrence Higgins Trust (1991) Statement on Sexual Health, cited in P. Aggleton and M. Toft, *Young People, Sexual Health and HIV/AIDS*, London, Health Education Authority.

Watney S. (1987) *Policing Desire: Pornography, AIDS and the Media*, London, Methuen.

Weeks, J. (1986) *Sexuality*, London, Tavistock.

Weil, A. (1986) *The Natural Mind*, Boston, Massachusetts, Houghton Mifflin.

Weiss, R. (1993) How Does HIV Cause AIDS? *Science*, 260, 5112, 1273–1279.

WHO (1987a) *Report of the Consultation on International Travel and HIV Infection*, Geneva, WHO, Global Programme on AIDS.

WHO (1987b) *Concepts of Sexual Health, Report of a Working Group Convened by the World Health Organization (EURO), 5–7 May 1987*, Copenhagen, World Health Organization.

WHO Global Programme on AIDS (1992a) *Current and Future Dimensions of the HIV/AIDS Pandemic: a Capsule Summary*, Geneva, WHO, Global Programme on AIDS.

WHO (1992b) *AIDS: Over a Million New Infections in Eight Months*, Press Release WHO/9, 12 February.

WHO (1992c) *Guide to Adapting Instructions on Condom Use*, Geneva, World Health Organization, Global Programme on AIDS.

WHO (1993) *The HIV/AIDS Epidemic: a Capsule Summary*, Geneva, World Health Organisation.

Wilton, T. (1992) *Antibody Politic: AIDS and Society*, Cheltenham, New Clarion Press.

Index

Acquired immune deficiency syndrome
see AIDS; HIV and AIDS
ACT UP, 45, 47
Age of consent, homosexual, and HIV
  education, 76
AIDS
  in Africa, WHO definitions, 29
  epidemiology, 56–60
    global, 57
    United Kingdom, 57–60
  HIV direct cytopathicity theory, 24
  independence loss fear, 99–100
  medical consequences, 99–101
  pathogenesis, 23–25
    theories, 24–25
  research priorities, 46–47
  science and medicine
    information/advice sources, 46
    keeping abreast, 45–46
AIDS and Drug Misuse, Part 1 (ACMD, 1988), 93, 95
Alcohol consumption, and safe sexual
  practices, 87
Alternative therapies, 44–45, 109–110
  legitimacy, 50–51
  risks, 44–45
Amphetamines, 88, 89, 90
Antibodies
  B cell, 16
  enhancing, 40–41
  neutralising, 40, 41
  see also HIV antibody test; HIV
    antibody-positivity
Anti–HIV interventions, 36–37
Antiretroviral drugs
  development, 33–35
  as early intervention, 37
  resistance, 37
  as symptomatic treatment, 37
Antiviral drugs, development
  difficulties, 20
α-APA compounds, reverse
  transcriptase inhibition, 36, 40
Apoptosis, 25
ARC (AIDS-related complex), 31
Artificial insemination by donor, HIV
  transmission, 85
Autoimmunity, 25
AZT (zidovudine), 31, 36, 37, 40
  and CD4(T4) cell count, 34, 38

β_2-microglobulin, and disease
  progression, 26
B lymphocytes (B cells), 15–16
  antibodies, 16
Bacterial opportunistic infections, 28
Bereavements, 103
Bisexuality, 78–79
  HIV and AIDS, 78–79
  see also Gay/bisexual men
Black/minority ethnic communities,
  safer sex, 83–84
Blood/blood products, HIV
  transmission, 62, 98
Body fluids/tissues
  HIV isolation, 60
  HIV transmission, 59
Body Positive groups, 7
Brain Committee (drug dependency),
  89–90
Breastfeeding, HIV transmission, 62–63
Buddy/befriender system, 107, 110
  and carer respite, 112

INDEX

Candida albicans, 28
Cannabis, 88, 89
Carer respite, and buddy/befriender services, 112
Caring and carers, 103
Case-control studies, 55
CD4(T4) cell count, 24, 30
 and AZT (zidovudine), 34, 38
 and disease progression, 26
CD4(T4) cells, 17, 41
 gp120 binding, 21, 23
 T cell syncytia, 24
CD4(T4) receptors, 21
 blocking, 36
CD8 cells, 16–17, 41
 HIV-infected, 25
Cellular immune response, 41
Centers for Disease Control (CDC) (USA), HIV infections stage definitions, 28–29
Cervical cancer, HPV-induced, 30
Children, of HIV-positive parents, 103–104
Children Act, 4
Citizens' Advice Bureaux (CAB), 111
Clinical trials
 access to, area differences, 107
 community consultation, 50
 design, 48–49
 representation/accessibility, 49
Cocaine, 88, 89
Cohort studies, 55
Coming to terms, 105–106
Community care, 7, 108–109, 110
Community Care Act (1992), 108, 110
Community drug teams (CDTs), 92
Community research groups, and treatment/research, 45–46
Compassionate Use programme, for treatment, 47
Complementary therapies, 44–45, 109–110
 legitimacy, 50–51
 risks, 44–45
Condoms, 80–82
 correct use, 81
 failure rate, 82
 female, 80
 and oral sex, 80–81
Contraceptive pill, and sex risks, 79
Council of Europe, travel and HIV testing statement, 69

Counselling, 112
 post-antibody testing, 67
 pre-antibody testing, 66–67
Crack cocaine, 90
Cryptococcus neoformans, 28
Cryptosporidium, 28
Cytokines, 25
Cytomegalovirus (CMV), 28

d4T (stavudine), 36
Dance drugs, 88, 90
Dangerous Drugs Acts (1920; 1923), 89
ddC (zalcitabine), 36, 40
ddI (didanosine), 36, 40
 MRC trial, 49
Defence of the Realm Act, Regulation 40B (1917), 89
Delay, and sex risk, 79, 80
Dendritic cells, HIV-infected, 25
Denial, and sex risk, 79
Dental dams, 81
Dental equipment, disinfection failure, and HIV, 63–64
Deoxyribonucleic acid (DNA), viral, 18, 20–21
Diagnosis, larger centres/local services, 107
Disabled people, and safer sex, 82–83
Discrimination, 8–9, 102
Displacement, and sex risk, 79–80
District nurses, 110
Drug dependence units (DDUs), 89–90, 92
Drug dependency
 development, 91
 maintenance therapy, 90
Drug development
 cautious optimism, 35
 difficulties, 20
 laboratory studies/human studies, 33–34
 mass media understanding and hype, 33, 34–35
 pace and structure of system, 35
 poorly conducted studies, 34
 provisos, 33–35
Drug use
 in Britain, history, 89–90
 diversity, 90–91
 mental/physical function effects, 91
 related problems, 91–92

Drug users
  attitudes to, 88–89
  HIV risk reduction/drug harm
    minimisation, 94–95
  negative attitudes to and beliefs,
    88–89
  specialist services, 92–93
  see also Injecting drug users
Drugs
  attitudes to, 88–89
  clinical trial design, 48–49
  negative attitudes to and beliefs,
    88–89

Ecstasy, 88, 90
Education, 113
Emotional support, 112
Endemic diseases, 54
Epidemics, 54
Epidemiology, 53–60
  data sources, 53–54

Family breakdown, drug-induced, 91
Family effects, of HIV/AIDS,
  104–105
Family Planning Association, sexual
  health definition, 72
Fc receptors, 41
Femidom, 80
Financial services, 111–112
Friendships, effects of HIV/AIDS, 104

Gay men's organisations, HIV victim
  support, 2
'Gay scene', 76
Gay/bisexual men
  HIV education targetting need, 59
  vulnerability to HIV/AIDS, 98
Gender, definition, 75
gp120, 21, 23, 41
  and AIDS pathogenesis, 24
  antibodies against, 36
GP fundholding, HIV care effects, 109
Granulocytes, 14, 15
Griffin Project (Turning Point), 93

Haemophiliacs, blood products and
  HIV/AIDS vulnerability, 98

Health education
  campaigns, 3
  training and learning needs, 5–6
  Health of the Nation, and injecting drug
    users, 94
Hepatitis B, 79
Heroin, 88, 89
Herpes, 79
Herpes simplex (HSV), 28
Herpes zoster, 28
Heterosexism, 76
Heterosexual men, safer sex, 84
Heterosexuality, 77–78
  stereotyped relationships and reality,
    77–78
High-risk groups, 3, 55
HIV, 17
  AIDS causation, 23–25, 27
  CD4(T4) receptor binding, 21, 23
  core protein p24 antigen, 26
  dormant state, 23
  epidemiology, 56–60
    Scotland, 58
    United Kingdom, 57–60
  first identification, 1
  immune cell destruction theory,
    24–25
  and immune system, 21–23
  life cycle, 21–23
  medical consequences, 99–101
  mutations, 25
  non-transmission situations, 63
  progression, 100–101
  social consequences, 101–106
  structure, 21
HIV and AIDS
  discriminatory attitudes/practices,
    8–9
  education
    facilitator-participant style, 8
    mainstreaming, 73
    monitoring/evaluation, 9–10
    needs assessment, 5–6
    participation/collaboration, 6–8
    and personal attitudes, 8
  local authority services, 2–3
  personal attitudes/beliefs, 4
  professional attitudes, 3–4
HIV antibody-positivity, 1
  emotional responses, 99
HIV antibody test, 64–65
  aims, 65–66

HIV antibody test (contd)
  confidentiality, 67—68
  false positive/false negative, 65
  post-test counselling, 67
  pre-test counselling, 66—67
  and travel/immigration, 68—69
HIV antigen test, 65
HIV centres, 107, 110—111
HIV infection
  progression
    and cofactors, 25—26
    and social groups, 26
    tests, 26
  risk factors, 55—56
  as a spectrum, 31
  stage definitions, 28—31
    debates, 29—30
    women's concerns, 30
  WHO official figures, 1
HIV Prevention Coordinators, as
  purchasers or providers, 108
HIV testing, 64—68
HIV transmission, 12, 19, 23, 56, 60—64
  artificial insemination by donor, 85
  blood and blood products, 62
  conditions, 61
  injecting drug users, 92, 93—94
  medical situations, 63—64
  mother to child, 62—63
  proven routes, 61
  sexual, 60
  and vaccines, 42
Homophobia, 85
Homosexuality
  and HIV infection, 2
  self-respect and sexual health, 85
  see also Gay men; Lesbians and gay
    men
Hospices, 107, 110
Housing, 99—100, 112
HTLV-1 (human lymphotrophic virus
  type 1), 20
Human immunodeficiency virus see
  HIV
Human papilloma virus (HPV), 28
  cervical cancer induction, 30
Humeral immune response, 40—44

Immigration, and HIV antibody testing,
  68—69
Immune cells, suicide (apoptosis), 25

Immune response
  cellular, 14—16, 41
  humoral, 15—16, 40—44
  to HIV, strength/weakness, 42
Immune system, 13—17
  cells, 14—17
  and HIV, 21—23
  strengthening or restoring, 39
  structure, 14—17
Immunity
  cell-mediated, 16—17
  humoral, 15—16
  non-specific, 14, 15
  specific, 14—17
Immunogens (therapeutic vaccines), 39
Immunostimulants, 39
Immunosuppression
  (immunodeficiency), 13
Incidence, of disease, 54
Independence, fear of loss, 104
Injecting drug users, 87—95
  drug-related problems, 92
  equipment sharing risks, 92, 93—94
  fears for children, 103—104
  HIV seroprevalence, 87—88
  and HIV transmission, 92, 93—94
  and needle exchange schemes,
    58—59
  social networks, 106
  vulnerability to HIV/AIDS, 98
Isospora belli, 28

Kaposi's sarcoma (KS), 27, 29, 56, 100
Killed vaccines, 43

Lassa fever, 54
Legionnaire's disease, 54
Lesbian and gay sexualities, 75—77
  and suicide, 76
Lesbians and gay men
  sense of self, 77
  sexual health, 84—85
Living with HIV and AIDS, 97—114
Local authority services, HIV and
  AIDS, 2—3
LSD, 88, 89, 90
Lymphocytes, 14—17
  clones, 15
  see also B lymphocytes (B cells); T
    lymphocytes (T cells)

Macrophages, 14, 15
Mainliners (drug user support/advice), 93
Medical care, 109–110
Medical consequences, 99–101
Medical situations, HIV transmission, 63–64
Memory cell responses, 41–42
Memory cells, 17
Meningitis, cryptococcal, 29
Methadone, 90, 92, 95
Misuse of Drugs Act (1971), 89, 91
Moralising, and HIV/AIDS, 105
Morbidity statistics, 53–54
Mortality statistics, 53–54
Mother to child, HIV transmission, 62–63, 103–104
Mycobacterium tuberculosis, 28

National AIDS Manual, 113
National Curriculum, 4
Needlestick injuries, HIV transmission, 63
Neopterin, and disease progression, 26
Nevirapine, 36
NHS
  reforms, 108–109
  staff, HIV testing guidelines, 68
  trust hospitals, and HIV services, 108
Non-governmental organisations (NGOs), HIV and AIDS education, 1–10
Nucleoside analogues, reverse transcriptase inhibition, 36, 40

Opiate dependence, 89–90
Opium. 89
Opportunistic infections, 13, 27, 28
  prophylaxis, as early intervention, 38
  treatment/prevention, 37–38, 100
Oral sex
  condom use, 80–81
  and HIV, 60
Organ transplants, HIV transmission, 62

Parallel Track programme, for treatment, 47
Pathogens, 14

Pelvic inflammatory disease (PID), 30
Pentamidine, aerosolised, PCP prophylaxis, 47
Personal identity, and HIV/AIDS, 105
Phagocytes, 14, 15
  antibody recognition/digestion, 16
Pneumocystis carinii pneumonia (PCP), 38, 56, 66
  life-threatening, 100
  pentamidine prophylaxis, 47
Positively Women, 7
  drug user support/advice, 93
Prejudice/discrimination, HIV/AIDS-related, 98–99, 101–103
Prevalence, of disease, 53, 54
Professional training curricula, and HIV and AIDS awareness, 3–4
Protease inhibitors, 37
  RT inhibitor combinations, 40
Protozoal opportunistic infections, 28
Proviruses, 19
Psychoses, drug-induced, 91
Public education, 102
Public health slogans, 97

Quality of life
  and AIDS, 98
  and community care, 110
  and complementary therapy, 44

Racism, 83–84
Recombinant vaccines, 43
Relationships, and HIV antibody-positivity, 104
Research, urgency, 47
Residential rehabilitation houses, and drug abuse, 93
Retrospective studies, of disease, 54–55
Retroviruses, 20–21
  life cycle, 20–23
Reverse transcriptase (RT), 21
  inhibitors, 36, 40
    combinations, 40
    protease inhibitor combinations, 40
Ribavirin, false hopes, 34
Ribonucleic acid (RNA), viral, 18, 20–21
Rimming, 82
Risk factors, and disease, 54–56

Risk groups, 55–56
Rolleston Committee (1926) (heroin prescription), 90

Safer sex, 2, 80–85
 and alcohol consumption, 87
 black/minority ethnic communities, 83–84
 and disabled people, 82–83
 emotional acceptance, 104
 heterosexual men, 84
 see also Sexual health
Saliva, HIV inhibition, 61
Salk HIV-immunogen vaccine, 43
Scat, 82
Self-blame, and self-esteem, 102
Self-esteem, and self-blame, 102
Self-help groups, 106
 and treatment/research, 45–46
Seroconversion, 64–65
Service provision, 106–113
 urban and rural differences, 107
Sex
 definition, 75
 and risk, 79–80
 sexuality and sexual behaviour, 75–79
Sex toys, 82
Sexual behaviour, 75–79
 change encouragement, 2, 3
Sexual health, 71–85
 concept, 71–73
 educator challenges, 74–75
 lesbians and gay men, 84–85
 power and scapegoating, 74–75
 and racism, 83–84
 sexual behaviour/desire diversity, 72–73
 see also Safer sex
Sexual identity, fluidity, 78
Sexuality
 disclosure, and HIV antibody-positivity, 105
 lesbian and gay, 75–77
Sexually transmitted diseases (STDs), 12, 79
Social consequences, 101–106
Social Fund, 111
Social work training, HIV and AIDS, 3
Street agencies, non-statutory, drug user advice, 92

Subunit vaccines, 43
Suicide, lesbians and gays, 76
Support groups, and services, 106–113
Synthetic vaccines, 43
Syphilis, 79

T lymphocytes (T cells), 16–17
 cytotoxic (CD8 cells) see CD8 cells
 helper (CD4/T4 cells) see CD4(T4) cells
tat inhibitors, 40
3TC (lamivudine), 36
Terence Higgins Trust, 7
 sexual health definitions, 72
TIBOL, 36
Toxoplasma gondii, 28
Travel, and HIV antibody testing, 68–69
Treatment
 and care
  access to, 47–48
  marginalised groups, 48
 combined interventions, 39–40
 expectations, 100–101
 geographical variations, 48
 minimum standard formulation, 48
 strategies, 36–40
 and trials, debates, 46–51
Treatment and Data Committee, New York, 47
Treatment IND, 47
Turning Point, Griffin Project for drug users, 93

Vaccines, 17
 preventive
  progress, 44
  prospects, 40–44
  safety, 42–43
  types, 43
 therapeutic, 39
Viral opportunistic infections, 28
Viral RNA, conversion to viral DNA, 20–21, 23
Viruses, 17–21
 activation, 20, 23
 reproduction, 19
 species-specific, 19
 structure, 18
 transmission, 19